Psychological Care in Practice

Psychological Care in Nursing Practice

Michael E Hyland
BSc, PhD
Senior Lecturer in Psychology
Plymouth Polytechnic

Morag L Donaldson
MA, PhD
Senior Lecturer in Psychology
Plymouth Polytechnic

SCUTARI PRESS

© Scutari Press 1989

A division of Scutari Projects, the publishing company of
the Royal College of Nursing

First published 1989

British Library Cataloguing-in-Publication Data

Hyland, Michael
    Psychological care in nursing practice.
    1. Medicine. Nursing. Psychological aspects
    I. Title. II. Donaldson, Morag
    610.73′01′9

    ISBN 1 871364 04 3

Printed in Great Britain at the Alden Press Oxford London and Northampton

Contents

Preface

In writing this book, we have been guided by many qualified and student nurses who have taught us about nursing while we, more formally, were teaching them about psychology. In learning about nursing we realised that much nursing is actually applied psychology. However we also found that, to teach psychology to nurses, it is necessary to use the nurse's perspective on psychology rather than the psychologist's. These two points underlie the organisation and selection of the content of this book. Its central message is that psychological care is crucially important to patients and their relatives, and that the nurses who provide effective psychological care are highly skilled professionals. This text is intended for nurses at all levels of training and experience who wish to develop skills in applied psychology that are intrinsic to nursing practice.

The material which is included in *Psychological Care in Nursing Practice* has been carefully selected. Our aim has been to write a book where psychology is included only to the extent that it relates to nursing practice. At the same time, we have tried to treat the psychological theory in sufficient depth to allow the student to obtain a critical awareness of the subject matter.

After an initial 'attitude orientation' chapter, the early chapters deal with basic aspects of communication. Later chapters deal with more complex aspects of communication and understanding, for example individual differences, caring for children and caring for the elderly. Yet later chapters cover topics such as pain, dying, bereavement and psychological aspects of physical illness. The topics covered in the different chapters are often interrelated and we have adopted the policy of putting the more general topics towards the beginning of the book. The book is intended to be read sequentially as later chapters build on material covered in earlier chapters.

In order to develop a critical research awareness in the reader, we give references to other people's work. We use both primary sources (i.e. the original research reports) and secondary sources (i.e. books or review articles which summarise the original research reports). When discussing general psychological principles which underlie a particular aspect of nursing we refer mainly to secondary sources. However, where there is research material which bears directly on nursing practice we refer to the primary research report. The primary sources are nursing as well as psychological journals. Both primary and secondary sources can be used as a guide to further reading.

In the text we have adopted the convention of using the masculine pronoun, 'he', for a patient (unless an example indicates to the contrary) and the feminine pronoun, 'she', for a nurse. This convention has been adopted in the interests of simplicity of writing style and, although we do not support the sexism it implies, we cannot reach an ideal solution. We apologise to anyone who may feel offended.

We hope you enjoy studying this book and that your learning will help maintain and develop the vital skills of the important profession of nursing.

Michael Hyland
Morag Donaldson

Acknowledgements

Many people have helped in one way or another in the preparation of this book. We give a list of their names below in alphabetical order. Those who have given most help know who they are and we give them a special thanks. There are many people whose names do not appear on this list, including our students, who have given their time and knowledge to help us write this book, and we are grateful to them too. We especially wish to mention Anne Blackburn, Mary Billing, Chris Frapwell, Susan Hinchliff, Sandra Hyland, Rosemary Morris, Margorie Oliver, Shaune Parker, Lyndsay Pearce, Elizabeth Parsons and Mary Watts.

1

Introduction to
Psychological Care

The aim of this book is to help nurses to develop psychological skills for that unique and crucial caring relationship with the patient which should occur in nursing practice. The insights so gained should form a basis for improved patient care as well as giving nurses increased pride and satisfaction in their important role.

The book has been written for nurses with advanced psychological skills just as much as for those who need to develop these skills. For the learner nurse, this book describes the skills which are necessary for providing psychological care. For the nurse who has already developed skills in psychological care this book provides the scientific evidence in support of those skills which she automatically employs. The skilled nurse can use this evidence to educate other nurses and support her own good practice in the face of possible criticism. By providing scientific evidence for good practice, it is the aim of this book to foster critical awareness of nursing practice.

For any nurse, however skilled, there is always room for improvement both in skill and in the knowledge base which underpins that skill.

The care which is provided by nurses is of two sorts:

1. Physical care
2. Psychological care

Physical care involves helping the patient to satisfy physical needs which, for one reason or another, he is unable to satisfy for himself. The help given by the nurse includes changing dressings, washing and feeding, giving injections and monitoring body functions. Psychological care involves looking after the patient's psychological needs, for example providing him with information about his condition and a sense of security and comfort.

Psychological care is very important to the patient. Psychological suffering can be just as real to him as physical suffering, and the skilful nurse can alleviate psychological difficulties just as she can alleviate physical ones. However, there is a second reason why psychological care is important. A patient's psychological state can radically alter the onset and course of physical illness, and a skilled nurse can use psychology to maintain and improve a patient's physical health.

The use of psychological care is also important for nurses. Providing psychological care means focusing on patients as people. People are interesting; people are appreciative; people are humorous; people are affectionate. Nursing is about people: that is one of its greatest attractions.

People vary in their ability to understand and relate to others. Some nurses have a natural ability: they automatically listen, observe, empathise and communicate well. Most health care professionals, however, need to develop these skills. It is not easy while learning the intricacies of a physical task—changing an intravenous infusion, managing a ventilator, remembering to give someone a bowl for washing their hands after using a bedpan—to see the person who needs care. Seeing the whole person comes with conscious practice and with the intention to include psychological care as a necessary part of the routine of nursing. The nurse who develops her psychological skills in nursing has the added reward of finding those skills useful in other contexts.

THEMES OF PSYCHOLOGICAL CARE

Each of the chapters in this book focuses on a different aspect of psychological care. However, there are certain themes which occur in more than one chapter. These themes are:

1. The holistic model of care
2. Communication
3. Differences between people
4. The right to self-determination and control

Holistic model of care

There are two models of disease which affect the practice of medicine and nursing: the *biological model* (also referred to as the *medical model*) and the *holistic model*. From the perspective of the biological model, disease is a purely biological phenomenon: for example, illness may be caused by the invasion of the body by bacteria or by physical degeneration of body tissue. From the perspective of the second model, however, disease must be understood holistically, that is, biological, psychological and social aspects of illness are all taken into account. There is now considerable research evidence in favour of the holistic model.

Holistic care is emphasised in two ways in this book. First, there is research (e.g. Jemmott and Locke, 1984) showing that a person's psychological state can radically alter the onset and outcome of an illness, i.e. disease is not a purely biological phenomenon, and the psychological aspects of care can have important consequences for the physical outcome of an illness.

Second, holistic care must be considered in terms of the patient's family. Relatives have psychological needs and can experience psychological suffering just as patients do. Relatives influence patients and patients affect relatives. Holistic care involves caring for the family as a whole.

Communication

Communication is crucial for effective psychological care because communication is the key for its achievement. Throughout this book suggestions are made about what to say—and what not to say—and ways of saying things. Two general topics of communication are discussed early on in the book. Chapter 2 focuses on ways of talking to clients in order to achieve a good therapeutic relationship. The quality of the therapeutic relationship is important for the success of many nursing actions, such as assessing the patient or helping to control his pain (see chapter 7). Chapter 3 covers ways of providing information so that patients maximise their self-care. Later chapters show how the basic principles of communication are altered to suit the circumstances of particular patients, for example the elderly, children and those who are dying or bereaved.

Differences between people

Each person requires a particular, unique form of nursing care and patients need to be communicated with and cared for in different ways to suit their particular needs. One implication of the differences between people is that nurses need to develop the skill of assessing people: they need to be able to form an impression of a patient's personality and to assess the way he reacts to particular types of situation.

In order to provide professional care for all their patients, nurses should be non-judgmental about the way patients choose to live their lives, particularly when the patient's life-style is rather different from their own.

Self-determination and control

Self-determination is a basic human need and right. It is the ability to choose a course of action for oneself and act on that choice. For example, nurses choose nursing as a career. Individuals choose whether they are going to smoke, to drive a car or go on holiday. To respect the dignity of an individual, the patient's right to self-determination must be allowed and assisted. One aspect of self-determination is the ability to look after oneself or be looked after in the way one wants. The patient's need for self-determination should, as far as possible, be respected by nursing and medical staff.

Nursing theory recognises the importance of self-determination through the concept of a *therapeutic contract*. When implementing a therapeutic contract, a nurse does not simply decide by herself what type of care is most suited to the patient. She advises the patient so that the form of care selected is based on a discussion between an informed patient and the nurse. A therapeutic contract implies that the patient retains a sense of self-determination and still feels in control of what is happening.

Self-determination is not the same as self-care. *Self-care* means that the patient cares for himself and, in the long term, self-care is an important objective. In the short term, however, nurses may need to provide the care which the patient is unable to provide for himself. For self-determination the patient decides the level of self-care he needs throughout his illness. There may be wide differences in how much self-care a patient wants to engage in: some patients prefer to look after themselves completely, whereas others prefer more help and nursing care.

Self-determination also implies that the patient's preference for the style of his care is respected. An extreme example of this is found in a style of nursing called 'therapeutic pampering' (MacStravic, 1986). In therapeutic pampering the patient's wishes come first. For example, the patient can have a bath when it is convenient for him, rather than at a time convenient for the ward staff.

Each of the four themes in this book (holistic care, communication, differences between people and self-determination) is intuitively reasonable. However, self-determination is a little less easily acknowledged, particularly when nurses are engaged in the hurly-burly of ward life.

Respecting the patient's self-determination can be problematic for two reasons. First, both patients and nurses have a need for self-determination and control. The nurse, like any other employee, likes to control what happens at work. However, the more the nurse controls what happens to a patient, the less the patient himself is in control of what happens. Thus, there can be a conflict between the nurse's and the patient's needs for self-determination. When caring for someone, it is easy to do too much.

Second, some patients tend to engage in self-harming behaviour, and their preferred style of care will not be conducive to good health. Overdependence, overindependence and other issues relating to self-harm will be considered in the book's final chapter.

The remainder of this chapter provides an introduction to some of the themes which will be developed later in the book, beginning with some of the basic research relating to self-determination.

LEARNED HELPLESSNESS THEORY

What happens to people when they are helpless? What happens when they are not in control of their environment? Seligman (1975) and his associates set out to answer these questions in the following way. One group of individuals was exposed to a controllable unpleasant event—a loud noise which could be turned off by pressing a button. A second group was exposed to an uncontrollable unpleasant event—a loud noise which could not be turned off at will but which stopped of its own accord. The researchers ensured that the second group of subjects received as much of the unpleasant event (the loud noise) as the first group. Individuals in the 'controllable' group and the 'uncontrollable' group were then given a second task, that of solving anagrams, and their ability to do this was measured. On average, people in the 'uncontrollable' group solved fewer anagrams than those in the 'controllable' group.

This and subsequent research led to a theory, called *learned helplessness theory*. It is called this because it deals with what happens when people learn that they are helpless, and cannot control what happens. Four different psychological phenomena can occur under conditions of helplessness.

1. *Cognitive deficit*: Problem-solving ability is reduced; people are less able to find solutions to new problems and less able to adapt to new situations. The cognitive deficit is a 'thinking' deficit.

2. *Motivational deficit*: Activity and the desire for action is reduced. The motivational deficit is a 'wanting' deficit.

3. *Sad affect*: People feel and appear depressed.

4. *Low self-esteem*: People feel worthless, of little value.

These four psychological changes do not always appear immediately. Under conditons of 'uncontrollability' many people go through an initial stage of *reactance* when they try and fight back and regain control. People who are reacting against uncontrollability do not suffer the above deficits, but may appear angry and hostile. Even if people are helpless for a period of time, deficits of helplessness do not necessarily occur. What matters is not whether people are actually helpless, but whether they think they are, and what they think has caused their helplessness (Abramson, Seligman and Teasdale, 1978). The psychological changes they suffer depend on answers to questions such as:

- How long is the cause of helplessness likely to last?
- Is the cause of helplessness due to me or to others?

This illustrates an important psychological characteristic which we shall return to more than once. It does not matter what the real or objective situation is: it is the subjective situation which actually affects people. It does not matter that there really are no ghosts; if one thinks there are ghosts, one's heart beats faster.

Attributions

The word *attribution* is a psychological term meaning 'the perceived cause of an event'. The attributions of helplessness are, therefore, the perceived causes of helplessness and these determine whether or not psychological deficits result from the experience of helplessness.

If a person believes that he is helpless because of his own deficiencies, then the above deficits, in particular sad affect (i.e. the feeling of depression) and low self-esteem are more likely to occur. For example, if someone is helpless and believes he is helpless because he is weak and stupid, then he is more likely to become depressed than if he attributes his helplessness to other people or to some aspect of the current situation. Psychologists distinguish *internal* attributions (where the person blames himself) from *external* attributions (where the person blames someone or something else). Research (Abramson, Seligman and Teasdale, 1978; Hyland, 1987) shows that people who blame themselves for things which go wrong suffer more psychological deficits than those who blame others. Interestingly, the people who blame themselves tend to be more accurate in their judgment but are more depressed. Under conditions of 'uncontrollability' it seems better to be happy and inaccurate than accurate and depressed.

Whether or not the attributions for lack of control are long-term or short-term can also affect whether helplessness deficits occur. If people think that their helplessness is of only a short duration they are less likely to develop the psychological deficits (cognitive and motivational deficits, sad affect and (low self-esteem) than if they believe helplessness will last.

To summarise, learned helplessness theory states that being in a state of helplessness can be bad. Not everyone exhibits psychological deficits under conditions of uncontrollability. Whether or not these deficits occur depends on whether the person perceives the cause of his situation to be internal or external (i.e. whether he blames himself or others) and whether it is short-term or long-term.

Although most of the research on learned helplessness has dealt with situations where helplessness has unpleasant consequences (e.g. a loud noise), other research (Winefield, 1983) examines the effects of helplessness leading to pleasant consequences. An example of helplessness leading to pleasant consequences would be where one is given money irrespective of one's actions. The research shows that even when the consequences are pleasant, helplessness can lead to psychological deficits.

It is sometimes easy for nurses to 'take control' of a patient so that pleasant consequences occur irrespective of what the patient wants or does. Ill health can, of course make patients helpless—that is, in some cases, its nature—and the nurse has to provide care which the patient cannot achieve for himself. But the nurse should not force the patient to be more helpless than he actually is, and she should be sensitive to day-to-day changes in the level of his helplessness. Some researchers (e.g. Raps, Peterson, Jones and Seligman, 1982) argue that 'hospitals are unpleasant places to be, in part, because they require patients to forfeit control which in turn results in various deficits'. That is, a style of caring where the patient's right of self-determination is removed by the nurse 'doing things' to the patient is, in fact, psychologically unpleasant. Patients may respond to such care either by reactance where, in the short term, the patient becomes hostile and tries to regain control, or, in the long term, by developing the psychological deficits associated with learned helplessness.

Raps et al (1982) argued that if hospitals did indeed reduce a patient's sense of control, there should be a gradual increase in the level of psychological deficit during a period of hospitalisation. They measured cognitive ability by assessing anagram-solving performance of hospital inpatients. The subjects were male, had an average age of 39 years, and none had a life threatening illness: The majority had orthopaedic complaints and the remainder had vascular and other problems. The patients' cognitive ability was measured regularly during their stay which, on average, lasted 11 weeks. They found that cognitive ability decreased throughout the 11-week period of hospitilisation. Raps et al also found an increase in depressed mood over the same period. Thus, the hypothesis that hospital care can induce helplessness and psychological deficit is supported by research.

Implications of learned helplessness for nursing

Imagine what it must be like to be an elderly person in some institutions. His basic needs are taken care of. Food is chosen for him. Dressing and bathing may be organised to suit the staff. He may be immobile. Whether pleasant or unpleasant things are happening, he may have little control.

It is hardly surprising that under such a 'caring' regime the elderly person may exhibit the cognitive and motivational deficits which can be hallmarks of institutionalisation. Furthermore, the elderly person, who may have been a useful member of the community before, now perceives himself to be useless and of no value. The lowered ability to think, the reduction in 'wanting' and the lowered self-esteem can be common features amongst the institutionalised elderly. This institutionalisation does not only occur with elderly patients – though it is far too often found in this context – but also can occur in any area of patient care. Nurses, too, can learn to be helpless; for example they may aim to be sensitive to the needs of others but may be prevented from being so by the organisation or leadership of the ward.

It should be noted (as discussed above) that not all patients exhibit helplessness deficits when placed in uncontrollable situations. A patient is more likely to show such deficits if he believes his helplessness to be long term (e.g. 'I am in here for the rest of my life') and also if he gives the situation an internal attribution ('I am helpless because my body has become so useless that I cannot help myself') rather than an external attribution ('I am helpless because that's the way this awful institution works'). Some patients may respond initially to uncontrollability with reactance. Patients who rebel and are labelled 'difficult' by the staff may not develop deficits, although they may experience other psychological problems.

Think for a moment how a 'naive' approach to nursing relates to learned helplessness theory. According to this naive approach, the nurse does things to the patient. The patient sits back (or should sit back) and accepts it gratefully, secure in the knowledge that nurses and doctors know best. The implication of this approach is that the patient should be helpless, or at least that the 'good' patient should be helpless. In fact, research (Kelly and May, 1982) shows that difficult patients are those who rock the boat by trying to intervene in their treatment. The 'unpopular' patient is one who fails to accept the sick and dependent role expected by nurses (Kelly and May, 1982; Stockwell, 1972).

- Nurse Armstrong is about to engage in a procedure which the patient is perfectly capable of doing himself.
  Patient to nurse: It's all right, dear. I can do that myself.
  Nurse: Don't worry. I am paid to do it. You just sit back and rest.

The point is that, although many people are attracted to nursing because it demands kindness, kindness without psychological knowledge does not necessarily lead to good psychological care. By 'being kind' to patients and doing everything for them, it is possible to have an effect which is detrimental to their well-being.

If kindness is combined with an understanding of a patient's own psychological needs, the patient is, as far as possible, actively involved in decisions relating to treatment. The patient and nurse agree a therapeutic contract. The nurse may encourage the patient to engage in self-care where appropriate, but the level of care and self-care is decided by the nurse and patient together, and is frequently reviewed. This means that the patient is no longer a helpless bystander in the process of care and treatment. The patient feels that he has some control over his care and treatment, which is what counts. A good nurse not only lets the patient participate but also communicates to him that he is participating.

Although most patients do like to have some control over what happens to them, there are times (for example, after shock or trauma) when people actually prefer or need to be cared for as though they are helpless. The extent to which a patient wishes to become dependent is an important personality characteristic which should affect the planning of care. Some patients accept or seek a helpless role, which may have detrimental effects on their health (see chapter 9); others react against the dependency and lack of control which their illness or care forces upon them. If the nurse respects the patient's right to self-determination she must also recognise his wish to be helpless.

DOES INDIVIDUALISED CARE HELP THE PATIENT?

A ward can be managed in different ways leading to differences in the way nurses and patients interact. A useful distinction is between *individualised care* and *task-oriented care*.

In task-oriented care, each nurse does one task for all the patients. A good analogy of task-oriented care is a car production line where one man only puts on wheels for all cars.

In individualised care, on the other hand, one nurse does all tasks for a particular patient, and is in a better position to get to know that patient. Individualised care is like the 'craft' approach to car production where a team is responsible for making a car from start to finish. Wards can be managed on a mixture of individualised and task-oriented care. For example, some nursing tasks might be done on a ward round basis but others on a patient-by-patient basis.

Primary nursing is an ideal form of individualised care. In primary nursing one nurse, the *primary nurse*, has 24-hour seven days-a-week responsibility for the care of a patient. When the primary nurse is not on duty, another nurse, *the associate nurse*, follows the general plan of care devised by the primary nurse.

Individualised care, and in particular primary nursing leads to a better relationship between the nurse and patient as the patient is able to get to know and trust one nurse and the nurse is, therefore, in a better position to provide psychological care. For example, a nurse who gets to know a patient will be less likely to 'take control' and induce feelings of helplessness, will be better able to communicate with the patient and better able to understand that patient's particular needs (Miller, 1984). The question remains, however, 'Does it make any difference?' Is there any evidence that individualised care or primary nursing is better than task-oriented care?

Miller (1985) compared elderly patients from two different types of ward: wards which were run on an individualised-care basis, and wards run on a task-oriented basis, which she called 'traditional' wards. Miller assessed the patients on several measures of dependency and also recorded the number of deaths and the numbers of patients discharged. She found no difference in the level of dependency between the two wards for short-term patients, that is patients who were in hospital for less than a month, but there were differences in dependency for long-term patients, that is patients in hospital for more than an month.

The differences in dependency (and characteristics of helplessness) for the long-term patients were striking. For example, 9 per cent of patients were in bed during the day in the individualised-care ward, but 45 per cent were in bed in the traditional ward. Thirty per cent were incontinent of faeces in the individualised-care ward, as opposed to 63 per cent in the traditional ward. Four per cent needed spoon-feeding in the individualised-care ward, compared with 16 per cent in the traditional ward.

In this study, Miller also examined the nurses' behaviour in the traditional and individualised-care wards. In the traditional wards, nurses had to 'batch process' a number of patients (about 30) and the patients' needs were subordinate to getting the task done quickly; consequently, nurses did not have time to relate to individual patients. In the individualised-care wards, between six and eight patients were allocated to a nurse. Patients were spoken to more often than in the traditonal wards. They were supported and educated to take care of themselves, and the nurses encouraged patient activity.

Miller also measured the numbers of deaths and discharges from hospital. Again there were differences between the individualised-care and traditional wards for long-stay patients, there being fewer deaths and more discharges in the individualised-care ward. Previous research (e.g. Brauer, Mackeprang and Bentzon, 1978) showed an association between dependency and mortality and so, if individualised care reduces dependency, it is not surprising that it also reduces mortality.

Miller concludes:

● 'In view of the association between traditional nursing, high patient dependency and lower discharge rates it cannot be emphasised too strongly that traditional nursing practices are positively unhealthy for elderly, long-stay patients. Since individualised care is associated with lower patient dependency, a shorter hospital stay, and a slightly better chance of surviving the hospital stay, and a slightly better chance of surviving the hospital stay, it does appear to have marked advantages.' (1985, pp.67–68)

The study also illustrates that wards are, indeed, managed in different ways. It can be quite difficult for a student to adapt from a task-oriented to an individualised-care ward and vice versa. In additon, the ward sister or charge nurse often believes that the way he or she is managing the ward is the correct way, and any other way is wrong.

Given that Miller's research shows clear advantages of individualised care, it is necessary to consider why some nurses prefer task-oriented care. The major advantages of task-oriented care are that it appears to work faster in the short term and that it is easier to ensure that essential care is given to all patients. The production line method of producing cars is indeed much faster than the craftsman approach—which is why most cars are produced that way. Similarly, if an elderly patient is having difficulty feeding himself, it is quicker for the nurse to feed the patient, than to help the patient feed himself.

But people are not cars. Caring for someone in a particular way actually alters the person. Although task-oriented care is undoubtedly quicker in the short term, in the long term it can increase work-load by increasing patient dependency. It can easily be seen how much more dependent were the long-stay patients in Miller's task-oriented wards, and how much more nursing care was, therefore, needed.

Not only are wards run on the basis of task-oriented or individualised care or some mixture of the two, but also ward sisters and charge nurses differ in their relative emphasis on psychological care. Although some people believe psychological care to be of paramount importance in nursing, and that in the long run time thus invested is time well spent, that view is not universally held or understood, and in some cases it may be felt that psychological care should always be secondary to the more pressing needs of physical care. There may be practical dilemmas for the student nurse in transit, but opportunities to promote an environment of holistic care can be realised when the nurse is qualified.

SUMMARY

This chapter introduced some of the basic ideas for providing psychological care. Psychological care is important to both patients and nurses. For the nurse, providing such care is a particularly rewarding aspect of her job. For the patient, psychological care reduces his psychological suffering and can enhance his physical recovery; research reviewed in this chapter demonstrates that the style of nursing employed is important to the patient's physical outcome.

Four themes appear throughout this book:

1. The holistic model of care
2. Communication
3. Differences between people
4. Self-determination

These different themes were introduced in this chapter, though an emphasis was placed on the need for self-determination. In particular, research on learned helplessness theory and the deficits associated with helplessness were discussed.

The opportunity to engage in psychological care is affected by the management of the ward. It is easier to provide psychological care in circumstances where individualised car is practised and in particular where there is primary nursing. However, whether or not psychological care is provided depends ultimately on whether the nurse wants to provide psychological care. Nursing is a profession, not just a job. The aim of the following chapters is to teach the basic ground-rules which a nurse can use to develop her own expertise in psychological care, and to show why psychological care is an essential part of good nursing.

References

Abramson L Y, Seligman M E P and Teasdale J D (1978) Learned helplessness in humans: critique and reformulation. *Journal of Abnormal Psychology*, **87**: 49–74.

Brauer E, Mackeprang B and Bentzon M (1978) Prognosis of survival in a geriatric population. *Scandinavian Journal of Social Medicine*, **6**: 17–24.

Hyland M E (1987) Control theory interpretation of psychological mechanisms of depression: comparison and integration of several theories. *Psychological Bulletin*, **102**: 109–121.

Jemmott J B and Locke S E (1984) Psychosocial factors, immunologic mediation, and human susceptibility to infectious diseases: how much do we know? *Psychological Bulletin*, **95**: 78–108.

Kelly M P and May D (1982) Good and bad patients: a review of the leterature and a theoretical critique. *Journal of Advanced Nursing*, **7**: 147–156.

MacStravic R S (1986) Therapeutic pampering. *Hospital and Health Services Administration*, **31(3)**: 59–69.

Miller A (1984) Nurse/patient dependency–a review of different approaches with particular reference to studies of the dependency of elderly patients. *Journal of Advanced Nursing*, **9**: 479–486.

Miller A (1985) Nurse/patient dependency–is it iatrogenic? *Journal of Advanced Nursing*, **10**: 63–69.

Raps C S, Peterson C Jones M and Seligman M E P (1982) Patient behavior in hospitals: helplessness, reactance, or both. *Journal of Personality and Social Psychology*, **42**: 1036–1041.

Seligman M E P (1975) *Helplessness: On Depression, Development and Death*. San Francisco: W H Freeman.

Stockwell F (1972) *The Unpopular Patient*. RCN Research Series. London: Royal College of Nursing.

Winefield A H (1983) Cognitive performance deficits induced by exposure to response-independent positive outcomes. *Motivation and Emotion*, **7**: 145–155.

2

Forming a Therapeutic Relationship

The moment the nurse steps on to a ward, into a health centre or into a patient's home, she will be communicating with people. Whether or not she wants to, she will be sending out messages, messages which go to patients, to other nurses, to doctors, to relatives, in fact to whoever is there. Communication is not an option. Once the nurse starts speaking, she sends information to these different people, and it is absolutely essential that she sends the right messages.

To be an effective communicator, the nurse must be able to send the right messages to other people and she must be able to read other people's messages correctly. This chapter concentrates on just one aspect of communication: how to form a good therapeutic relationship.

A therapeutic relationship is a feeling of trust and understanding between two people. Anyone can have a therapeutic relationship with another person. For example, parents often have therapeutic relations with their children, which is one reason why it is important to involve parents in the care of hospitalised children (see chapter 6). However, for the nurse, a therapeutic relationship is a professional tool which she uses to achieve nursing objectives relating to psychological care, such as alleviating pain, giving information and aiding physical recovery. Two basic skills help to form a therapeutic relationship:

1. Giving people the message that the nurse cares for and likes them, and understands how they are feeling

2. Reading the messages that others are sending, to understand their needs, feelings and thoughts

   This chapter is organised in three parts.

1. *Non-verbal communication*, or 'body language', consists of the ways in which people send messages using signals other than spoken or written words. These signals include, for example, posture and facial expression.

2. *Verbal communication* consists of the messages which are put into words. The account of verbal communication given in this chapter is restricted to how it is used to develop a therapeutic relationship; information-giving and other aspects of verbal communication are covered in later chapters.

3. *Emotional recognition* is the skill of using verbal and non-verbal signals to discover the emotional experiences of another person.

NON-VERBAL COMMUNICATION

Non-verbal communication has three functions (Argyle, 1975).

1. It communicates feelings about other people, for example a nurse can use non-verbal communication to show a patient that she likes him. If the patient thinks he is liked he will tend to reciprocate these feelings.

2. It acts to support verbal communication. Correct use of non-verbal communication helps reinforce verbal communication between nurse and patient and shows the patient that the nurse is interested in what he is saying.

3. It provides a replacement for verbal communication when verbal communication is not possible. Even when verbal communication is possible, a gesture or touch sometimes says more than words.

COMMUNICATING FEELINGS

People seldom tell others outright whether or not they like them, but almost all the time people send out non-verbal messages which tell others how they feel about them. This happens in four main ways:

1. Eye contact
2. Pupil size
3. Facial expression
4. Body posture

Eye contact

Research by Exline and Winters (1965) shows that a person looks more at someone who is liked than at someone who is disliked. Moreover, there is more eye contact (when two people look each other in the eye) between people who like each other than between people who do not. So if a nurse does not like a patient her natural inclination will be to avoid looking at him and to avoid eye contact. To put it differently, people usually interpret a nurse's looking at them and eye contact as a sign of liking.

A person may avoid eye contact for a number of reasons: he may be depressed, embarrassed or simply shy. Unfortunately, when someone avoids eye contact this signal is usually interpreted as dislike rather than depression, embarrassment or shyness. A nurse who feels shy should make a special effort to look patients in the eye. Likewise, patients may also be shy or embarrassed, so the fact that a patient avoids eye contact with a nurse does not necessarily mean that he dislikes the nurse.

Argyle (1975) found that when two people are talking, each person spends about 60 per cent of the time looking at the other and about 30 per cent of the time having eye contact. However, the amount of 'looking' and eye contact depends very much on the context. Therefore, to signal liking someone, one must have the right amount of 'looking' and eye contact for the context. Some of the factors which affect the normal level of eye contact are listed below.

Gender

Females tend to engage in more 'looking' and eye contact than males. In particular, female–female eye contact is much higher than male–male eye contact.

Distance

The amount of looking and eye contact depends on the distance between the two individuals: the further one is from someone, the more one looks at them.

The reason why a person looks less at others in close proximity is that eye contact can be physiologically arousing, particularly at such short distances. In many social contexts, moderate levels of arousal are pleasant but high levels of arousal are uncomfortable (Apter, 1984). Think about what happens when people are forced to stand close to each other in a lift: everyone looks at the floor or at the indicator numbers and so avoids eye contact.

However, where there is a strong loving bond between two people, high arousal can be enjoyable, which explains why lovers are happy to stare closely into each other's eyes. Nurses should not have an intimate relationship with patients and so should reduce eye contact when engaging in a procedure which involves close face-to-face proximity.

Culture

In Middle Eastern and Latin cultures the normal amount of eye contact is much higher than in that of Western Europe. On the other hand, American Indians have lower levels of eye contact than Europeans; in their social system looking someone in the eye can be interpreted as a sign of disrespect. The historical stereotype of a 'shifty-eyed Indian' is one result of this culture clash—the Red Indian's lack of eye contact was interpreted by the white settlers as dishonesty. When communicating with someone from a different cultural background, it is important to make allowances for the different non-verbal style of that culture.

Hostility

Eye contact, in most social contexts, indicates liking, but there is an exception. In situations of extreme hostility, eye contact means strong dislike. If a nurse is caring for a patient with a known history of violence who starts staring at her, she should be on the alert for an aggressive outburst. In situations of extreme tension and hostility, reduction in eye contact is to be recommended. This will reduce the other person's physiological arousal and thereby reduce the confrontational nature of the interaction.

The physiologically arousing effect of eye contact means that its amount should not be excessive. Staring (that is, an amount of eye contact which is too great for what is normal in a particualr context) is interpreted as aggressive, intimidating, intrusive or simply bizarre.

The nurses's objective should be to maintain a reasonably high level of 'looking' for the particular situation. Obviously, an intuitive judgment is needed about the optimum level of eye contact, and one way to gauge this is to take the cue from the patient. The more he looks at the nurse, the more she should return the look, and vice versa. A patient who is avoiding eye contact should not be forced into a response. Eye contact is a mutual interaction which requires adjustment by at least one of the people interacting, and that person should be the nurse and not the patient.

Pupil size

The pupil is the black hole in the iris, the coloured area of the eye. It is well known that the size of the pupil is affected by the light level, but pupil size is also affected by physiological state (opiate, drugs, for example, constrict the pupil) and by feelings for a person. 'Liking' tends to dilate the pupil, whereas 'disliking' leads to constriction.

That pupil size is an indicator of positive feeling was known centuries ago in China. Merchants selling jade ornaments would hold a prize piece behind their back and then suddenly show it to a prospective customer: the price went up if the customer's pupils dilated!

Hess (1972) took two identical pictures of a smiling girl and painted larger pupils onto one of the pictures. When men were presented with the pictures and asked which one they preferred, all selected the one with enlarged pupils. They reported that the girl was smiling more which, of course, was inaccurate. Interestingly, this effect disappears if homosexual men are questioned.

Little can be done to alter pupil size, although the drug belladonna (the Italian word for 'beautiful lady') was used as an early cosmetic to dilate pupils. It is worth remembering, however, that a nurse may find herself disliking people receiving opiate drugs (which are used as analgesics) simply because they have constricted pupils.

Facial expression

Common sense tells us that facial expression should be a good indicator of like or dislike of a person. To a certain extent, this common sense assumption is true (Ekman, Sorenson and Friesen, 1969). Smiling is almost always interpreted as liking, and is a good signal to send, even if one does not feel much like smiling.

On the other hand, smiling is not a reliable signal that someone is happy or that he likes the person at whom he is smiling. In general, interpreting patients' feelings from their facial expressions can be unreliable for two main reasons.

First, people tend to express emotions in ways which are unique to them. Facial expression communicates much about the feelings of somebody one knows well, as one is likely to be familiar with how that person's face reflects their emotions. However, if someone is not familiar, it is easy to misinterpret feelings by relying on facial expression. Misinterpretation of smiling is exacerbated for people who have had cerebrovascular accidents or suffer form Bell's palsy. In Parkinson's disease facial muscles have an unnatural immobility which can be misleading.

Second, some people hide their emotions by presenting a 'conventional face'. That is, they show facial expressions on the basis of what they think is conventionally required rather than what they are actually feeling. Commonly this takes the form of 'putting on a brave face' or 'keeping a stiff upper lip'. We all know that the face is used to communicate emotions so we modify our expressions to hide our feelings.

It is important to remember that there are differences in the way people express emotion. Some people tend to smile more than others, whereas others are perfectly happy but do not naturally smile. If a patient is not smiling, he may still be happy and like the nurse. Conversely, if a patient is smiling, he may just be putting a brave face on his unhappiness. Thus, the nurse must be careful not to jump to wrong conclusions on the basis of facial expression.

Body posture

Another way by which people communicate their feelings is in the distance they stand from others. People tend to stand closer to those whom they like, and further from those whom they do not like. Again, the 'normal' distance one person stands from another is affected by context; for example people from Middle Eastern and Latin cultures tend to stand much closer to each other. There are, in fact, training schemes for businessmen who are going to the Middle East to teach them to stand close to their host and look him in the eyes so that they do not appear unfriendly.

The way in which people sit is also an important indicator of how they feel about someone else. A *closed posture* (see figure 2.1) is adopted indicating that social interaction is not wanted. On the other hand, an *open posture* indicates willingness to interact. It is sometimes appropriate for the nurse to sit on a patient's bed or on a chair by the bed to reduce interpersonal distance. If the nurse then wishes to cross her legs, she should ensure that the leg furthest from the patient is crossed over the leg nearest to the patient, and that the body is orientated towards the patient, thereby achieving an 'open' stance.

Suppose one is going to sit with someone at a square table. Should one sit opposite them or at 90 degrees? The answer depends on the kind of relationship desired. Sitting opposite someone tends to be interpreted either as competitive and confrontational or as intimate. Sitting at right angles tends to be interpreted as cooperative. In most nursing contexts, and particularly when visiting patients at home, the signal of cooperation rather than competition is required, so sitting at 90 degrees is to be preferred. Incidentally, during interviews, the 'chair straight opposite the desk' postion is perceived to be less friendly than the 'chair at the side' position.

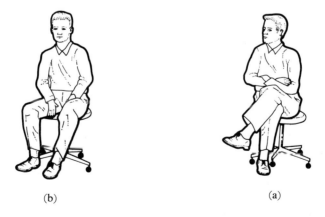

(b)   (a)

Fig. 2.1 (a) Closed posture, (b) Open posture.

SUPPORTING VERBAL COMMUNICATION

Non-verbal communication can support verbal communication by showing participants when to take turns during a conversation and by indicating the listener's interest in what is being said.

1. *Taking turns*: Non-verbal signals are used to tell others when a person is about to start and stop speaking (Argyle, 1975). Of course, these signals are not essential for conversation to take place (people can talk just as effectively by telephone) but they can be a substantial aid to verbal communication. When the speaker is coming to the end of what he is saying, he then looks at the listener. This look is a signal meaning 'it's your turn now'. On the other hand, a person who is about to start speaking signals his intention to do so by looking away: this means, 'It's my turn now'. The nurse can use eye contact to encourage someone to speak. The nurse who says, 'How are you feeling, Mrs Jones?' while looking at the thermometer sends the message that she is not interested in Mrs Jones' answer.

2. *Showing interest*: There are four non-verbal signals which show that the listener is interested in what is being said. First, by maintaining eye contact, the listener sends the signal, 'Keep going, I am not going to interrupt'. Second, nodding the head at the end of statements indicates interest, but these head nods should not be random. When head nods are synchronised with the other person's speech, they are an important way of giving the message, 'I understand what you are saying'. Rapid head nodding, however, can signal, 'Yes, I know, and I want to interrupt'. Third, 'Mmm' or 'Uh-hu' responses indicate interest. Again these noises should be synchronised with the other person's speech so as to come at the end of important statements. Fourth, emotion should be *reflected*. Reflecting emotion means portraying the kind of emotions that the other person is showing. For example, if the speaker is reporting something which is distressing, the listener should mirror the distress.

The above four points add up to something which is called *active listening*. When listening to what a patient is saying, the nurse must not sit passively: she should actively listen, which means attending to what the other person is saying and sending the correct non-verbal signals in response. Active listening requires effort and practice.

REPLACEMENT OF SPEECH

Sometimes speech cannot be used in communication, for instance with the deaf. Patients suffering some types of brain damage can hear and understand but cannot speak. Under these circumstances, non-verbal signs can be used to replace speech. Some deaf people use elaborate sign languages (such as British Sign Language and American Sign Language) but for patients who do not know these languages communication is still possible.

The nurse should first try to find out the capabilities and limitations of the patient who has a communication handicap and then try to find some way of overcoming the difficulty. Many such patients will be able to recognise objects and point to pictures of them. The use of pictures (the nurse can draw them herself, they do not need to be works of art) is an important aid to patients suffering from communication difficulties.

Even if the patient can hear and speak, non-verbal communication is sometimes more effective than words. The nursing action of *presencing* (Benner, 1984) occurs when a nurse is simply near a patient. Presencing can provide reassurance as well as alleviating the lonelines which can occur when a patient is seriously ill or in acute pain, such as the pain of labour.

Touch can also be used to communicate with patients. It is useful to distinguish between *instrumental* touch, i.e. touch which occurs during a nursing procedure, and *expressive* touch, i.e. touch which is used to express emotions (Porter, Redfern, Wilson-Barnett and Le May, 1986). Expressive touch, such as a light touch on the arm, is a good way of showing understanding and appreciation of how the patient is feeling.

However, there are conventions about using expressive touch in Western cultures, where touching is less acceptable than in, for instance, Latin cultures. Female–female physical contact is much more common than male–male physical contact (Henley, 1973). Hoffman (1972) found that female patients reacted more positively to touch than males, but that men would accept physical contact, particularly if they were under stress or very old (Watson, 1975). However, irrespective of gender, some people are naturally more 'touchable' than others.

When deciding whether or not a patient will welcome expressive touch, the nurse can be guided by research carried out by Whitcher and Fisher (1979). These researchers observed the effect of nurses touching or not touching patients during preoperative preparation using several indices: patient satisfaction with information given, blood pressure and how much of a preoperative leaflet was read. Women showed greater satisfaction, displayed lower blood pressure and read more if touched, but the reverse was found with males. The authors interpret these findings by hypothesising that touch can imply that the touched person has a dependent (helpless) role. Men react more negatively to adopting a dependent role and therefore, in this study, reacted negatively to touch.

Whether or not someone accepts a dependent role depends on their personality as well as their physical condition. A general rule to follow is that most people appreciate expressive touch in times of crises because, at such times, a dependent role is more often sought. However, the nurse should avoid expressive contact with those who are responding to hospitalisation with reactance behaviour (i.e. showing anger and demanding information) as these people will resent the dependency role that touching implies.

Research shows that touching or stroking the skin can have the important effect of inducing relaxation, with measurable physiological consequences. For example, Lynch et al (1974) found that physical contact (such as holding a patient's hand) can affect the patient's heart rate and reduce the frequency of ectopic heart beats, the irregular heart beats that may accompany heart attacks. Effective use of touch also leads patients to perceive the carer as being more competent (Blondis and Jackson, 1977). Other research (Lynch, 1977) shows that touching other people or even pets has a relaxing effect.

Of course, much nurse–patient physical contact is instrumental and is accepted as such by both male and female patients who see it as being part of the legitimate role of the nurse. However, it is possible for a patient to confuse instrumental with expressive touch, and such confusion is particularly undesirable when touching intimate areas of the patient's body. One way of avoiding confusion is for the nurse to inform the patient of what she is doing, and instrumental touch can also be carried out with reduced eye contact in cases where confusion could arise.

Non-verbal communication: implications for nurses

It is likely that many readers, having completed the preceding sections will think, 'I do that already'. What have been described in these sections are social skills, in which many people are competent. However, a person's ability to use non-verbal signals does vary quite widely.

Research shows that the extent to which health professionals are liked by patients is highly influenced by their ability to send friendly non-verbal messages (LaCrosse, 1975). Some carers have very poor social skills which leads to difficulty in their making friends. Someone who is shy, sits in a closed posture and avoids eye contact is sending out messages that he does not want to make friends, and this is often the case with lonely people. Help can be obtained through social skills training schemes which, in essence, teach a person by providing him with the information covered above and then making a video film of the trainee while he is interacting with others. When a person sees himself as others see him, and realises the sort of inappropriate non-verbal signals he is emitting, he is in a good position to start improving his non-verbal behaviour.

Even if a nurse is a skilled non-verbal communicator, there are certain circumstances when her social skills may not be at their best. By anticipating these difficult circumstances, it is possible to maintain a consistently high standard of communication when dealing with patients.

Fatigue

When tired, a person's natural reaction is to protect himself from the physiologically arousing effects of dealing with others. A tired nurse might protect herself by avoiding eye contact, maintaining a large physical distance between herself and the patient, and employing a closed body posture, everything, in fact, which gives the message that she does not like the patient. Thus, when tired it is necessary to make a special effort with regard to non-verbal communication.

Dislike of a patient

No nurse likes all patients, nor should she feel guilty about, or try to deny, disliking some of them. However, it is part of the role of a professional nurse not to show such dislike, and she must be especially aware of using the appropriate non-verbal signals in such circumstances.

Summary

Below is a list of the most important non-verbal signals which can be used to help form a good relationship with a patient, relative or fellow nurse.

1. High levels of eye contact (particularly when the other person is speaking or when the nurse is coming to the end of a statement or question) indicate liking and interest.

2. The use of head nods, 'Uh-huh' noises and emotional reflection indicate attention to and understanding of the other person's speech.

3. An open body posture and appropriate physical distance from the listener make a person more likely to talk freely.

4. Expressive touch can be a useful way of communicating sympathy and understanding, particularly when a patient or relative is at a time of crisis.

VERBAL COMMUNICATION

A nurse can use verbal communication to find out what others are thinking and feeling, and to give information. This section focuses on the 'finding-out' function of verbal behaviour, and is divided into five parts:

1. Open and closed questioning
2. Non-directive and directive questioning
3. Reflecting statements
4. Understanding coded messages
5. Exploratory responses and counselling

Open and closed questions

Closed questions are those questions which can be answered with the words 'Yes' or 'No'. For example, the question, 'Are you feeling better?' can be answered in this way.

Open questions cannot be answered with the words 'Yes' or 'No'. For example, the question, 'How are you feeling?' might produce the answer: 'I am feeling a lot better, thank you'.

Open questions:

● Elicit more conversation

● Are more likely to lead to spontaneously given information

● Require more effort on the part of the respondent

In general, open questions should be used rather than closed questions unless there are specific reasons for preferring closed questions. Closed questions, however, have an important role to play under certain circumstances.

● Closed questions should be used if simple factual information is needed, for example, 'Have you been to see your general practitioner about this?'

- Closed questions may be better when dealing with an elderly, confused patient who has difficulty answering. It is easier to reply to a closed question and the answer is less likely to be ambiguous.

- If a patient is in an acute phase of an illness, the extra effort required to answer an open question places an additional and unnecessary burden on the patient, and such patients do not necessarily want the extra responsibility that open questions impose on them. It is, therefore, sometimes better to ask closed questions when patients are highly distressed.

- If the patient is having breathing difficulties a closed question is easier to answer, and can be answered non-verbally, for example by a nod or shake of the head.

Directive and non-directive questioning

Whereas open and closed questioning refers to the actual questions asked, directive and non-directive questioning refers to the way an interview is structured, that is, how all the different questions fit together.

It is possible to organise an interview on the basis of certain specific predetermined objectives. For example, the nurse might want to find out about the patient's accommodation and whether anyone else lives there. Questions which are asked according to a predetermined plan are called *directive*. Alternatively, the nurse might not have specific predetermined objectives for an interview, but only a general idea of possible topics. If that is the case, she can employ an alternative style of questioning, called *non-directive*. In non-directive questioning (Rogers, 1951) the interviewer picks up on key words in what the patient has just said and asks for them to be expanded.

- *Nurse*: How are things at home?
  Patient: Well, we are having one or two problems.
  Nurse: What sort of problems?
  Patient: Mainly with my mother who is staying with us.
  Nurse: Uh-huh?
  Patient: Well, she doesn't get on with my son.
  Nurse: Why not?
  Patient: Well, . . .

Notice that after the first question the nurse is not directing the conversation in any way. The conversation is directed by what the patient thinks is important.

Non-directive questioning should be used to find out what is important from the patient's point of view. It is a useful way of satisfying the patient's rather than the nurse's, communication needs (Alfano, 1985). Directive questioning should be used to obtain information important to the nurse. Obviously, both sorts of questioning will have their uses at different times.

Reflecting statements

Reflecting statements have the effect of expressing sympathy with and understanding of the other person.

- *Nurse*: How did you feel last night?
  Patient: Well, it was pretty bad at times.
  Nurse: Had a bit of a rough night, did you?

What the nurse has done is rephrase what the patient has said. Reflecting statements are a very useful way of building up a positive relationship: they show that the nurse cares and understands what her client is feeling and thinking.

There can be a danger with reflecting statements in that the nurse misunderstands the patient and reflects something which the patient did not mean. Exploratory responses (see below) help detect bad misinterpretations and are sometimes preferable to reflecting statements, particularly when there is the possibility of ambiguity.

Reading coded messages

People sometimes do not say what they mean, but they often give a clue to what they really mean by sending a 'coded' message. Reading coded messages is a difficult skill and is something which has to be done intuitively. There are, however, some pointers to help in this area.

Jokes

Jokes almost always have a serious side to them and people will often make a joke of something about which they are extremely anxious. For example, a young man reporting chest pains may joke, 'I had better increase my life insurance cover' where what he really means is, 'Is it likely that I am going to die?' It is always worth paying good attention to patients' jokes.

Oblique questions

People sometimes ask questions which may provide the information they want without needing to ask the question outright. Faulkner (1985) gives the example of a patient who discusses with a nurse whether she should buy a pet dog. The real question being asked is, 'Will I survive to look after the dog if I buy him?'

The 'hand-on-the-door' phenomenon

People sometimes disclose their real worries as they are leaving the room or as the conversation is coming to an end. A classic example is the housewife who calls on a friend for coffee and on the way out says, 'Oh, by the way, my husband has just left me'. Statements made when the hand is (at least psychologically) 'on the door' are often presented in an incidental, not-very-important, manner. The nurse should pay attention to sudden shifts in conversation when a person is leaving, as this often signifies that he wants to discuss something but is having difficulty in doing so.

Overemphatic denial

When a denial is made for no apparent reason or if a denial is overemphatic, it may not be true. There is a line in Shakespeare's play, 'Hamlet', which illustrates this point: 'The lady doth protest too much, methinks' (*Hamlet*, III. ii. 242). Patients who shout, 'I am perfectly all right' or who suddenly say out of the blue, 'There is no problem between me and my wife' may, at some unconscious level, mean quite the reverse. Denials are a way of coping with threats to the individual's peace of mind which are barely conscious.

Projection

Patients sometimes project their own anxiety onto someone else. For example, a patient may say, 'My wife is very anxious about what is happening; I wonder if you could have a word with her', when it is actually the patient himself who is anxious.

Reacting to coded messages

The problem with coded messages is that they *are* coded, and it is difficult to tell whether one has cracked the code correctly. A good way of reacting to what appears to be a coded anxiety message is to provide reassurance (provided that reassurance is realistic).

If a nurse suspects that a coded message is being sent but is unsure of its meaning she should try, tactfully, to explore further. It is important to remember, though, that the reason the message was coded in the first place was because the patient does not want to make the message explicit, and the patient's wishes should be respected. With hidden messages, it is often best to give information or ask questions as though these come spontaneously from the nurse rather than as a response to what the patient has just said.

The patient may need time to 'uncode' the message himself before talking about something distressing. He should not be hurried: there are times when it is best for the nurse to say nothing. Understanding and responding to coded messages need tact and sensitivity.

- Mrs Stephenson was having a hysterectomy following a cervical smear test which showed malignant cells. Her sister had previously had a hysterectomy but later died of cancer. Mrs Stephenson was convinced she too was going to die of cancer but had not told anyone at the hospital about her sister. However, student nurse Miller heard Mrs Stephenson asking another patient, also about to undergo a hysterectomy, whether any of her relatives had had the operation. Student nurse Miller guessed that there might have been a reason for Mrs Stephenson asking the question and so asked her the same question a little while later. On finding out about Mrs Stephenson's sister, student nurse Miller was able to reassure Mrs Stephenson that cervical cancer does not seem to have a hereditary basis and that her sister's death would not alter her own chances of survival.

Sometimes coded messages reflect anxiety about the patient's feelings rather than the patient's condition. For example, people sometimes feel angry and resentful about a dying relative, and these feelings are themselves a source of distress. The nurse should provide reassurance by interpreting the emotion, for example, 'I am not surprised you feel angry. I know I would be absolutely livid. But you really are managing very well.'

Interpreting emotions in this way improves self-confidence at times when confidence-boosting is very important. It is absolutely crucial that the nurse does not deny the patient's or relatives' emotions, with statements like, 'Well, you will just have to pull yourself together' or, 'There is no reason for you to feel that way' or, 'This is just something you will have to come to terms with'. Nurses should try to help patients believe in themselves and give them reassurance. It is not appropriate to say, 'Don't worry, you will be all right.' The first stage in reassuring a patient is to reassure him that his worries are legitimate.

Exploratory responses and counselling

Because patients often have no-one else to turn to, a nurse may take on the role of counsellor. However, research (Hills and Knowles, 1983) does indicate that nurses often lack counselling skills.

Orlando (1961, 1972) has made a particular contribution to the study of the nurse's role as counsellor. On the basis of her observation, Orlando came to the conclusion that 'good' nurse–patient interactions were characterised by *exploratory responses* i.e. the nurse responds in ways which help both the nurse and the patient understand how the patient is feeling. The nurse should use tentative statements such as, 'If I understand you correctly . . .' or, 'What I feel you are trying to tell me . . .' and follow assertions with comments such as, 'Am I right?'. These exploratory responses can be contrasted with *declarative responses* which involve statements telling the patient how he is feeling.

Exploratory responses are related to the reflecting statements described above. According to Orlando, however, a reflecting statement should not simply be a declaration but should be followed by a question to the patient as to whether the reflection is, in fact, correct.

Exploratory responses encourage a constant feedback between the nurse and patient where the patient says something and the nurse asks a question to see if she understands correctly what the patient has said. Exploratory responses are therefore more likely to build up an accurate picture for the nurse of how the patient is feeling, rather than an inaccurate picture based on prior assumptions. The advantage of exploratory responses is that they help the patient feel cared for by the nurse, they encourage further conversation and disclosure on the part of the patient, and they help the patient to think about himself which can aid his recovery (see chapter 9).

Orlando's suggestions about how nurses should provide counselling support owe much to the ideas of Rogers (1951). Two of his concepts are *unconditional positive regard* and the *uniqueness of personhood*.

According to Rogers, counselling proceeds best in an atmosphere of unconditional positive regard, which means that the patient or client feels that he will still be liked by the counsellor whatever he says. Conditional positive regard, on the other hand, occurs where the counsellor only shows affection for the patient when the latter is saying the 'right' things. From a nursing perspective, unconditional positive regard means that the nurse should be non-judgmental when talking to a patient. If there are any judgments to be made, the patient should make them himself without bias from the nurse. Although it is very difficult to be non-judgmental (see chapter 4), unconditional positive regard is a goal to aim for when caring for patients. Appropriate use of non-verbal cues may help hide a tendency to be judgmental.

Unconditional positive regard is important to the patient because it helps him to talk about distressing events and express the emotion associated with these events.

Although there are occasions when patients express emotion which requires 'interpreting' by the nurse (see above), there are also occasions when patients do not know whether they should express emotion and unconditional positive regard helps to unlock these hidden emotions. Furthermore, as western culture often denies the free expression of emotion, the nurse may need to provide the patient with a sense of positive permission to express his feelings. A patient will recognise positive permission through exploratory responses as, correctly given, these indicate that the nurse is genuinely interested in what he is feeling.

Rogerian counselling is based on the idea that everyone is unique and that people should be allowed to develop in their own unique way. When providing counselling and advice it is important not to try to shift people away from their own unique way of existing to a way which the nurse thinks is better. This, ultimately, goes back to the point made in chapter 1, that people have a right to self-determination, and psychological problems can result if people are prevented from controlling their own destiny.

A useful summary of the aims of counselling is provided by Nichols (1984). These are:

1. To make the situation safe (without threat to the patient)
2. To enable the client to get 'in touch' with his feelings
3. Give permission for the expression of their feelings
4. To communicate understanding and empathy
5. To communicate acceptance of the patient
6. To share personal feelings with the client
7. To support the client.

The most frequent errors made by nurses in a counselling context are, first, not allowing the patient to express emotions (e.g. by saying to him, 'Don't worry, you will be all right) and, second, giving advice (albeit the correct advice) without allowing the patient time to express himself first.

Summary of verbal communication

This section has focused on the role of verbal communication in obtaining information from others. Five topics were discussed: (a) the use of open and closed questions, (b) the use of reflecting statements, (d) how to understand and respond to hidden messages, and (e) basic counselling skills and exploratory responses.

EMOTIONAL RECOGNITION

The ability to assess how another person is feeling is an important part of nursing. Emotions are private experiences but can be inferred from behaviour: from verbal behaviour, from non-verbal behaviour and from the interaction between the two.

People vary in their willingness or unwillingness to express emotions, often due to the way they have been brought up. For example, some people have been brought up to 'keep a stiff upper lip' and not show their mood. Others show their emotions to anyone and everyone. There is some evidence (see chapter 9) that the inhibition of spontaneous emotion can be harmful to physical health.

If a person is willing to express his emotions verbal communication is probably the most accurate way of assessing how he is feeling. Careful questioning and exploratory responses can lead to a picture of a patient's or relative's private world of experience. Problems in interpreting emotions arise if someone is unfamiliar with expressing, or unable or unwilling to express, emotions. In such a situation, the nurse can still make an assessment by monitoring *emotional leakage* (Buck, 1984). This is the term used for behaviours which 'leak out' and therefore show what someone is really feeling. Speech content is the least 'leaky' of the emotional signals, followed by facial expression: people know what to say and how to appear in order to indicate the emotion they wish to portray.

Other parts of the body are more 'leaky' than the face. In particular, excessive movements of the hands and feet indicate feelings of anxiety, discomfort or boredom. Tapping or shaking of the foot and drumming of the fingers are signs of discomfort.

Tone of voice is slightly more 'leaky' than the body. For example, a flat tone of speaking can indicate depression, whereas a staccato, high-pitched way of talking can indicate anxiety.

The most 'leaky' part of emotional behaviour is the relationship between the individual behaviours. Under normal circumstances, verbal and non-verbal communication mesh together, i.e. they 'fit' with each other. However, if a person is trying to conceal his emotions, the verbal and non-verbal behaviours no longer mesh. In reply to the question, 'How are you feeling?', a person who is feeling good will probably smile and then say, 'Fine'. However, a person who is trying to hide his sadness will first say, 'Fine' – and then smile.

The failure of non-verbal and verbal communication to mesh does not always indicate concealment. It may mean that that different parts of the person's mind are saying different things. For example, a person may have a conflict of goals between wanting to do something and not wanting to do it (see chapter 4). Under such circumstances, it is possible for the person to say one thing verbally and send the opposite message non-verbally. As a general rule, however, if verbal and non-verbal messages do not mesh the nurse should not take the verbal message at face value.

People will sometimes try to deceive about things other than emotions, for instance factual information. Although it is difficult to assess whether someone is hiding the truth, deception is often accompanied by an increased rate of blinking of the eyelids, and by a hesitation or pause before answering. However, it is very difficult to assess whether deception is taking place unless the person is well known as it is necessary to know the person's normal rate of these behaviours; some people blink and hesitate a lot under normal circumstances.

Dealing with people who are trying to deceive requires sensitivity on the part of the nurse. The nurse should not confront the patient with his deception, but should try to use unconditional positive regard to create an atmosphere where deception is unnecessary.

PUTTING THEORY INTO PRACTICE

A large number of skills have been discussed in this chapter, so many that it is difficult to grasp all the different details at once. Burnard (1985) suggests that nurses go through stages in learning to communicate: an *unaware* stage, an *aware* stage and a *skilled* stage (see also Benner, 1984). A nurse cannot expect to do everything correctly at first, so should not be discouraged if a conversation with a client does not go well. Realising that an interaction went badly is the first step to putting communication right.

The basic rules for establishing a relationship are that the nurse should attend to what her patient is saying and that she should treat him courteously as a person rather than as a body with an illness. Although this may seem obvious, research shows that nursing practice often falls short of these ideals. In a study of patient satisfaction with hospitalisation, Inguanzo and Harju (1985) found that 27 per cent of patients expressed some dissatisfaction with nursing care; of those expressing dissatisfaction, 36 per cent said the reason was 'discourteous nurses'. Thus, the old-fashioned idea of good manners is a useful focus for developing communication skills. It is sometimes helpful for the nurse to think of clients not as hospital patients but as guests, with her as their hostess.

Repeated interaction with patients should help to develop communication skills but it is not necessarily the case that experience in nursing improves communication. Sharkey (1985) suggests that many basic nurse training programmes are 'harmful to empathy and individuality'. This statement is backed up by the findings of Crotty (1985), who found that learner nurses communicated more with patients than did sisters or trained staff. A nurse will improve her communication skills only when she tries to do so and this requires commitment and effort.

SUMMARY

The purpose of this chapter has been to introduce some of the basic ideas and skills for forming a therapeutic relationship. In a therapeutic relationship a patient trusts the nurse and the nurse understands how the patient thinks and feels. This chapter has covered both the non-verbal and verbal behaviours which help form a therapeutic relationship. With regard to non-verbal behaviour, emphasis was placed on signals which show liking, interest and concern. For verbal behaviour, emphasis was placed on questioning, reflecting, exploring, and counselling. A final section of the chapter covered the recognition of emotion.

References

Alfano G (1985) Whom do you care for? *Nursing Practice,* **1(1)**: 28–31.
Apter M J (1984) Reversal theory and personality: a review. *Journal of Research in Personality,* **18**: 265–288.
Argyle M (1975) *Bodily Communication.* London: Methuen.
Benner P (1984) *From Novice to Expert.* Menlo Park, California: Addison-Wesley.

Blondis M N and Jackson B E (1977) *Nonverbal Communication with Patients.* New York: John Wiley & Sons Ltd.

Buck R (1984) *The Communication of Emotion.* New York: Guilford Press.

Burnard P (1985) Learning to communicate. *Nursing Mirror,* **161(8)**: 30–31.

Crotty M (1985) Communication between nurses and their patients. *Nurse Education Today,* **5**: 130–134.

Ekman P, Sorenson E R and Friesen W V (1969) Pan-cultural elements in facial displays of emotion. *Science,* **164**: 86–88.

Exline R V and Winter L C (1965) Affective relations and mutual gaze in dyads. In: *Affect, Cognition and Personality,* eds. Tomkins S and Izzard C. New York: Springer.

Faulkner A (1985) *Nursing: A Creative Approach.* London: Baillière Tindall.

Henley N M (1973) Status and sex. Some touching observations. *Bulletin of the Psychonomic Society,* **2**: 91–93.

Hess E H (1972) Pupilometrics. In: *Handbook of Psychophysiology,* eds. Greenfield N S and Sternback R A. New York: Holt.

Hills M D and Knowles D (1983) Nurses' levels of empathy and respect in simulated interactions with patients. *International Journal of Nursing Studies,* **20**: 83–87.

Hoffman L W (1972) Early childhood experiences and women's achievement motives. *Journal of Social Issues,* **28**: 157–176.

Inguanzo J M and Harju M (1985) Consumer satisfaction with hospitalization. *Hospitals,* **59(9)**: 81–83.

LaCrosse M B (1975) Nonverbal behaviour and perceived counsellor attractiveness and persuasiveness. *Journal of Counselling Psychology,* **22**: 563–566.

Lynch J J (1977) *The Broken Heart; Medical Consequences of Loneliness.* New York: Basic Books.

Lynch J J, Thomas S A, Mills M E, Malinow K and Katcher A H (1974) The effects of human contact on cardiac arrhythmia in coronary care patients. *Journal of Nervous and Mental Diseases,* **158**: 88–89.

Nichols K A (1984) *Psychological Care in Physical Illness.* Croom Helm.

Orlando I J (1961) *The Dynamic Nurse–Patient Relationship.* New York: Putnam's Sons.

Orlando I J (1972) *The Discipline and Teaching of Nursing Process.* New York: Putnam's Sons.

Porter L, Redfern S, Wilson-Barnett J and Le May A (1986) The development of an observation schedule for measuring nurse–patient touch, using an ergonomic approach. *International Journal of Nursing Studies,* **23**: 11–20.

Rogers C R (1951) *Client-Centered Therapy.* Boston, Massachusetts: Houghton Mifflin.

Sharkey J (1985) Learning not to understand. *Nursing Times,* **81(16)**: 50.

Watson W H (1975) The meaning of touch: geriatric nursing. *Journal of Community,* **25**: 104–111.

Whitcher S J and Fisher J (1979) Multidimensional reaction to therapeutic touch in a hospital setting. *Journal of Personality and Social Psychology,* **37**:87–96.

3
Giving Information

A nurse is better able to understand what a patient thinks and feels by listening to him and asking him questions. After having listened to a patient the nurse may judge it necessary to give him information and this chapter covers the topic of information-giving.

There are two major reasons why a patient may be given information. First, the patient wants or needs the information. Information is necessary for the patient to control what happens to him, and so the need for information is part of the more general need for self-determination. If he is (or suspects that he is) denied information he will react with feelings of anxiety.

The second reason for giving patients information is to promote self-care. Patients may need to care for themselves, or be cared for by relatives, both in hospital and in the community. Self-care requires information so, apart from her other duties, the nurse also has the role of teacher or health educator.

Although this chapter shows how a nurse should approach her role of information-giver, it is important to emphasise that information-giving must be combined with information-seeking on the part of the nurse. She should assess the patient's information needs before providing information; thus, questioning and information-giving are interrelated topics.

This chapter is divided into four sections. The first section gives an introduction to the topic of information-giving. The second section discusses how to explain things to patients in ways which help them to understand what is said. The third section discusses how to present information in ways which help patients to remember the information given, and the fourth section explains how to give information in ways which increase the likelihood that this information will be accepted.

INTRODUCTION TO INFORMATION-GIVING

If patients are questioned about their experiences in hospital, the most usual area of complaint is the dearth of information given. This lack of satisfaction with communication has been found in over 20 studies (see review by French, 1981) and, although the precise proportion varies between studies, it seems that about 50 per cent are dissatisfied with information given.

For example in an early study McGhee (1961) interviewed patients in their homes, 10 to 14 days after discharge from hospital. The area of greatest dissatisfaction with their stay in hospital was communication, and about 65 per cent expressed some dissatisfaction with this aspect of care. In a more recent study, Engstrom (1984) found that 41 per cent of patients reported that information about the likely outcome of their stay (the prognosis of their health problem) was 'entirely inadequate', 36 per cent found information about diagnosis to be 'entirely inadequate', and 19 per cent drew the same conclusion for information about after-care. Engstrom points out that these results were obtained despite the likely extra effort put into communication by staff who were aware that the study was being carried out.

Part of the lack of patient satisfaction with information has, of course, to do with other staff, e.g. doctors, but there are two reasons why nurses cannot be excused from responsibility for information-giving. The first is that nurses are in a unique position to give information, as the high level of nurse–patient contact enables the nurse to get to know the patient and to make sure that information is correctly understood. Second, research shows that nurses do not communicate well with patients, although other groups of hospital staff may have even worse communication problems. For example, Crotty (1985) observed nurses interacting with patients and concluded: 'The findings from this study suggest that verbal interaction by all grades of nursing staff is not satisfactory in either quantity or quality'.

Patients' opinions about nurses have also been studied using questionnaires (e.g. Inguanzo and Harju, 1985; Moores and Thompson, 1986) and these studies confirm Crotty's findings: patients perceive nurses to be too busy or too caught up in routine tasks to talk to them.

There are several reasons why nurses should try to ensure that patients are satisfied with the information which is given.

1. Dissatisfaction with information leads to anxiety, which is an unpleasant psychological state. Nurses should care for patients in ways which minimise psychological suffering.

2. The anxiety which results from lack of information can exacerbate pain (see chapter 7) and can interfere with good physical health (see chapter 9).

3. Satisfied patients are more likely to follow health care instructions (Dunbar and Agras, 1980; Ley 1982).

4. Satisfaction with information improves the patient's uptake of the health care services. Satisfied patients are less likely to delay seeking care when it is needed and are more likely to respond to symptoms (MacStravic, 1986). Satisfaction with information is therefore important for prevention of future ill health.

In general terms, then, a patient who is satisfied with information gets more health benefits than a dissatisfied patient.

Why are patients so often dissatisfied with information? This dissatisfaction results from the interaction between patients on the one hand and nursing and medical staff on the other.

First, medical and nursing staff often perceive communication to be of secondary importance to curative procedures and other care (Ley and Spelman, 1967) and, consequently, insufficient time is devoted to communication. Even where time is spent on communication, the information may not be presented effectively. Engstrom suggests that some nurses fail to 'individualise and adjust' the information they are giving; in other words, the information is put across in a way which is unsuitable for a particular patient.

Second, patients are often diffident about asking for information, particularly in distressing circumstances. Some patients feel intimidated or feel that, if they do ask questions, they will appear to be stupid. Patients may also feel reluctant to 'waste the nurse's time' by asking questions. Cartwright (1964) found social class differences in questioning behaviour in that patients who were in the professional class asked many more questions than patients who were partly skilled or unskilled workers.

So, in very general terms, communication difficulties arise because patients do not ask enough and because medical and nursing staff do not explain enough or explain properly.

The following sections deal with:

● Helping people understand what they are told
● Helping people remember what they are told
● Helping people accept what they have been told

IMPROVING UNDERSTANDING

Several factors must be taken into account when the nurse tries to help people understand the information she is giving.

The patient's understanding of illness

Any job has a special language which goes with it, and a nurse learns the special language which goes with nursing. It is easy for her to forget that medical and nursing terms are not part of other people's language, even though they are part of her everyday vocabulary. Clearly, using words which others do not understand will not help them to accept her information.

Ley and Spelman (1967) suggest that people can understand and follow straight forward instructions such as 'Stop smoking' or 'Rest for half an hour after meals'. However, they are less able to understand and follow instructions which contain even slightly technical terms. For example, people have difficulty in complying with the advice 'Avoid foods containing starch' or 'Avoid substances containing aspirin' because they often have incorrect notions (Riley, 1966) about which substances contain starch or aspirin.

Not surprisingly, people have difficulty with instructions which are potentially ambiguous. For example, an instruction given at a health centre to 'Phone up for an emergency appointment only when it *is* an emergency' is ambiguous because it is not clear exactly what constitutes an emergency situation.

Several studies have been carried out to find out how much patients understand of illness. Ley and Spelman (1967) found that although the majority of people did understand correctly about different illnesses, there was still a substantial minority who were ignorant about many aspects of illness. For example, Ley and Spelman questioned members of the public on their knowledge of diabetes and found that 40 per cent were ignorant of the symptoms, 15 per cent were ignorant of treatment, 19 per cent were ignorant of diagnostic procedures, and 37 per cent were ignorant of the outcome of the conditon. In fact, two subjects who were themselves diabetic thought that diabetes was diagnosed by taking the blood pressure. One wonders what they thought the constant urine testing was for! In the same study, Ley and Spelman found that 44 per cent thought that lung cancer is usually cured by treatment.

Not only are people ignorant about illness, but they are also often ignorant about human anatomy. Boyle (1970) found that 54 per cent of people did not know where their kidneys were, 50 per cent incorrectly located their stomachs, and 49 per cent did not know the positioning of their lungs.

It is useful to use non-technical terms, or to explain what technical terms mean, as a way of increasing patients' comprehension. However, as a first step it is important to find out what patients understand; some people may say that they understand something when they do not in order to avoid appearing stupid. Thus, sensitivity and tact is needed in questioning patients.

Some patients are knowledgeable about medical conditions. Interest in medicine is an important determinant of medical knowledge and seems to be related to the number of illnesses a patient has experienced (Ley and Spelman, 1967). The more knowledgeable patient is likely to have a greater need for information about his present condition, and the nurse should try to satisfy that greater need.

Distractions

To understand what he is being told, a person needs to concentrate on what is being said. In a noisy environment, attention wanders due to the distracting effect of noise. There are also internal distractions: if someone is very upset or in pain, he may not attend to what he is being told. It is best to give information in circumstances where there are few external distractions, and to avoid giving complex information when someone is very upset, in pain or when he may be otherwise distracted.

Distraction can occur if the client wants to find out something other than, or in addition to, what the nurse is telling him. Thus, the nurse should find out what the patient wants to know before launching into a monologue where she tells the patient what she thinks he wants to know. Information-giving should be accompanied by questioning or exploratory statements (see chapter 2) and should always be appropriate to the patient's needs.

A good way to check for distraction is to assess the level of eye contact. If the patient is looking around rather than maintaining eye contact he may not be listening to the nurse. However, eye contact may also be avoided for cultural reasons or because the person is embarrassed about the information being given.

Accent and grammar

Although the patient may speak English, there are different accents of English (based on region, class or ethnic background) and it cannot be assumed that the patient will understand the nurse's accent. Grammatical structure also differs; for example, some people are used to rather short sentences, whereas others are more accustomed to longer ones. It is useful for the nurse to listen actively to the way a patient speaks as a way of alerting her to possible difficulties of dialect and grammatical structure. Differences of accent are particularly likely to create communication problems if a patient has poor hearing which is particularly common in elderly patients (see chapter 5).

If the nurse suspects that a patient has not understood what has been said due to differences in accent, poor hearing or simply lack of attention, it is a good strategy for her to repeat the sentence exactly as she said it the first time. If the patient still does not understand, the sentence can be rephrased.

The overall strategy in helping people understand is to 'individualise' the information given to match both the patient's ability to understand and what he wants to understand. In order to match information-giving to the particular patient, the nurse should first assess the patient's communication needs: information-giving involves discussion where the nurse attends to and is sensitive to what the patient is trying to say.

HELPING PEOPLE REMEMBER WHAT THEY ARE TOLD

Even if patients do understand what they are told, they may not remember all of it. Ley and Spelman (1965) interviewed patients after they had seen a doctor, and compared the patient's recall of material with the written record kept by the doctor. Patients did not remember everything, and some information was less well remembered than the rest. Their findings are summarised in table 3.1.

It appears from this table that patients remember their diagnosis best, followed by details of further visits, and then information on their prognosis. Self-care instructions are least well remembered.

What are the factors which cause this lack of memory, and what can be done to prevent it? In particular, how can the nurse improve memory for self-care instructions?

Anxiety and embarrassment

Research (Humphreys and Revelle, 1984) shows that the ability to remember a fact gets worse with rising levels of anxiety. For example, a common experience is that of revising just before an examination and feeling that nothing is sinking in. The anxiety about the examination is probably preventing learning. Research in a hospital context confirms that a patient's ability to remember information is impaired by high levels of anxiety (Ley and Spelman, 1967).

To the nurse, the patient's arrival in hospital is routine and commonplace, but to

Table 3.1 Retention of information

Category of statement	Percentage statements recalled
Statements about diagnosis	86·5
Statements about treatment prognosis and explanation of symptoms	55·5
Statements about further visits and investigations	77·0
Instructions and advice	43·5
Other statements	30·0

the patient, going to hospital is never routine. Patients are often highly anxious, both on arrival and at medical consultations where they imagine they are 'going to learn their fate'. Although this anxiety may not be sufficiently great to prevent the patient understanding what he is told, nevertheless he may not remember it. It can be a useful strategy to check later that a patient has remembered the information he has been given.

Patients are often highly anxious when consulting a doctor or when spoken to on a ward round. Moreover, doctors do not always communicate adequately. Therefore, it is useful for a nurse to speak to a patient after the consultation, either to translate medical 'jargon' into easily-understood language, or to provide repetition of the same information under less anxious circumstances.

Embarrassment can also lead to poor retention of information, and embarrassed patients are also less likely to ask questions and offer comments. Cartwright gives an example of a young female patient who said after a ward round:

- 'I had a sort of a blank, you know, especially when you have five or six of them round you and when they're young, too, and you're stripped. You sort of dry up and don't know whether to say it or not, when there's two or three, in case they think you're soppy.' (1964, p.89)

Lack of sensitivity to a patient's feelings will always lead to poor communication and poor remembering of facts. A general policy should be to ensure that the patient is psychologically 'comfortable' to enhance his comprehension and memory. In practice this means that the nurse should select the time to give information on the basis of her assessment of the patient's psychological state.

Presentation of information

Psychological research shows that the order of presentation of items of information can affect what is remembered (Ley and Spelman, 1967). If a list of statements is read out to a person, he is more likely to remember the first few statements and the last few statements and forget the statements in the middle of the list.

If a patient is given information in a logical sequence, e.g.:

- What is wrong with him
- What he ought to do
- What is likely to happen to him

the middle statement, 'What he ought to do', is likely to be the most frequently forgotten (see table 3.1).

In order to increase the likelihood of the patient remembering health care instructions, the nurse can repeat her advice to the patient at the end of her list of statements, e.g.:

- What is wrong with him
- What he ought to do
- What is likely to happen to him
- What he ought to do

Not surprisingly, the more information that is given, the more the patient is likely to forget. If a substantial amount of information is to be given (for example three or more statements) it is essential that the patient has some written record to help his memory. The nurse should write the information down herself as she describes each item to the patient, and then give the written record to the patient to take away. Alternatively, the information can be typed after the interview. It should not, however, be assumed that every patient is able to read.

If a patient is being discharged with instructions about how to care for himself at home, it is important that the patient is given written material, even if he appears to understand what to do. Memory tends to be 'context specific', i.e. retention of information is more likely in the situation in which it was learnt. Even if the information is remembered once the patient is at home, the written record helps allay any anxiety about whether it was remembered correctly.

Organisation of information

Information is rembered best if it is presented in organised categories (Dunbar and Agras, 1980; Ley and Spelman, 1967). For example, a nurse can begin by saying, 'I'm going to start by telling you what we have found out about your condition', and then tell the patient what is wrong with him. She could end with, 'I want to tell you now what you ought to do when you go home, and this is very important for how quickly you'll get better', and then present the self-care instructions.

Notice how, in this example, the nurse has made explicit to the patient the type of information she is giving. When giving information, it is useful for the nurse to make sure that the order of presentation and categories of material are organised before starting the interview.

Importance of information to the patient

Psychological research also shows that the perceived importance of the information to the recipient affects whether it is remembered or not. Engstrom (1984) found that patients perceive diagnosis and prognosis to be more important than self-care instructions, and these findings are consistent with those of Ley and Spelman (1976) who found that patients remember self-care instructions least well.

When presenting self-care instructions, it is a useful strategy to stress to the patient that what you are saying is important to the eventual outcome.

Failure to carry out instructions

Sometimes patients remember what they have been told, but do not remember to carry out their self-care. They want to follow instructions but do not get round to doing so. This is a common reason for irregular use of medication; for example, many patients forget to take antibiotics as prescribed (Ley and Spelman, 1967). In some cases forgetting to take a drug at the correct time can be very serious: e.g. failure to take insulin can result in diabetic coma.

Memory aids can help patients to take medication correctly. For example if medication is linked with normally occurring events (e.g. 'Take one before meals') the patient is less likely to forget his tablets. Drugs can be placed where the patient is likely to find them on a regular basis (e.g. next to the toothbrush). Alarm clocks can be used to alert the patient to the fact that drugs should be taken and some modern digital wrist-watches have an alarm function which can be a helpful, and more discreet, alerting device.

Where multiple drugs are being taken and there is the possibility of confusion a useful strategy is to put all the drugs for that day into a cup (or series of cups) first thing in the morning. Alternatively, it is possible to mark when drugs are taken on a chart. Doing so avoids the 'Have I taken it or not?' question which, if answered incorrectly, can lead to over- or underdosing.

If appropriate, memory aids should be suggested at the same time as the nurse gives other self-care instructions, but it should be done in a way which is not patronising or insulting. For example, it is unhelpful to say, 'You are likely to forget to take these pills at the proper time, so set your alarm clock to remind you'. More appropriate is: 'It's ever so easy to forget to take these pills at the proper time. Some people find setting their alarm clock useful. That way they don't worry about forgetting. And it will help you get to better much more quickly if you take the pills on time'. The final sentence in this example gives a reason for taking the pills which is important to the patient's compliance, and this is something which is expanded on in the next section.

Summary

1. Memory is improved if the time and the situation in which information is given is carefully selected to ensure that the patient is neither highly anxious, embarrassed nor upset.

2. Memory of self-care instructions is improved if they are repeated at the end of an interview session and their importance stressed.

3. A written record helps memory and is particularly necessary if there are complex self-care instructions.

4. Material is better remembered when organised into categories.

5. Memory aids can help some patients remember material when they have gone home.

6. All patients experience memory problems at times. It is important to assist retention of information for all patients, not just those who seem likely to forget.

ACCEPTANCE OF INFORMATION

Many patients who understand and remember what a nurse tells them will also accept that information; after all, nurses are often perceived to be people in authority and to know what they are talking about. However, there are occasions when the patient will not accept what he is told and it is sometimes *because* the nurse is an authority figure that her advice and information are rejected.

There are two related reasons why a patient may reject the information which is given: because the information is personally threatening or because the information requires self-care actions which the patient does not want to carry out. The effects of these reactions can be reduced by skilful communication.

Personally-threatening information

Information may be rejected if it is too personally threatening to the patient, i.e. if it threatens his concept of his own self. For example, it is personally threatening for a patient to realise that his liver has been damaged by his own excessive intake of alcohol, or to find his body image changing after a colostomy. It is even more personally threatening for him to learn that he is dying, or for a mother to realise that the small size of her newborn baby is the result of her own smoking. Information may also be personally threatening to relatives who may learn that their care at home has been inadequate.

A frequent reaction to such information is outright denial. A person may deny that he is dying (see chapter 9); a mother may deny that smoking was the cause of her newborn child's problems. Extreme sensitivity is therefore needed in giving personally-threatening information, and the way the information is given is crucial to how and whether it is accepted.

There are three important rules in giving personally-threatening information.

1. The information should come from someone who has formed a therapeutic relationship with the patient and whom the patient trusts. An atmosphere of unconditional positive regard should be cultivated.

2. The information should be given only when the patient is ready and the nurse should assess this by talking to the patient. Some patients take longer than others to become ready to receive such information.

3. Although patients generally want information, they may not want personally-threatening information. The direct 'sledgehammer' approach may be less effective than a more subtle approach where the information appears to come from the patient himself.

The following two examples illustrate good and bad information-giving. Both examples relate to a similar type of situation, where a mother who has smoked heavily during pregnancy has a light-for-dates baby in a special care baby unit. It is worth bearing in mind that, given the media publicity regarding smoking and pregnancy, mothers who smoke during pregnancy are likely to have received information about the risks involved, and may also have a low regard for authority.

- *Dr J*: Now Mrs Ellis, the reason your baby is so small is because you smoked when you were pregnant, and I can tell you that if you smoke again during pregnancy your next baby will be just as small. (*Dr J exits*)
  Mrs Ellis (to nurse): Sod the doctor; I'm going to have a fag now.
  Nurse (thinks): I feel like having a cigarette too.

- Here the client and nurse have formed a good therapeutic relationship.
  Mrs Rogers: Do you think my smoking caused my baby's problems?
  Nurse: Well, what do you think?
  Mrs Rogers: I suppose it could have done.
  Nurse: Mm. They do say it can, don't they. What do you think?
  Mrs Rogers: Well, I suppose I shouldn't smoke next time.
  Nurse: I think you're probably making the right decision. After all, that way you're more likely to have a healthy baby.

There is a belief among some health-care professionals that accurate and unambiguous information should always be given, even if the patient does not want it. The above examples illustrate, however, that information should be given in a way which is acceptable to the patient. The 'sledgehammer' approach can lead to what can be called the 'Sod you' reaction. Patients may not say 'Sod you' to the carer's face but they can go away thinking it.

The second example shows how skilful the nurse was in giving information. She did not actually give the information but let Mrs Rogers work it out for herself. If the patient works it out himself he really does believe the facts, but when the information appears to come from the nurse, the patient will only believe it if it can be made consistent with his other beliefs.

Another feature of the second example is that the information was provided in an atmosphere of unconditional positive regard. The nurse did not give the impression that she was sitting in judgment on the mother as a person because of her smoking. A final feature of the second example is that the nurse waited for Mrs Rogers to be ready to accept information rather than forcing the issue like Dr J had.

The example below further illustrates the importance of choosing the right time for patient education.

- Mrs Wright (aged 54) is to have a hysterectomy. This is the first operation she has had. She is extremely frightened about the possibility of dying under the anaesthetic and is worried about not being 'a woman' when she loses her womb. Mrs Wright, who is a successful businesswoman, is also concerned about appearing incompetent and anxious.

Nurse: Would you like to know a little bit about the operation?
Mrs Wright (smiling inappropriately): No, no, don't bother; I'm fine.
Nurse (thinks): Let's give her time to settle down and then give her another go.
Later that evening when Mrs Wright is more relaxed:
Nurse: Have you had an operation before?
Mrs Wright: No. (*pause*) No.
Nurse: It must be all quite new to you.
Mrs Wright: Well yes. Really, I don't know what is going to happen at all.
Nurse: What would you like to know about?
Mrs Wright: Well the anaesthetic, for instance. Is it dangerous; does it always work?
The nurse then provides the relevant information (see chapter 7).

The nurse must always assess when a patient is ready to accept information which is personally threatening. Some people are always ready, others need time, and the nurse should treat patients according to their individual needs. Patients may indicate that they are ready for information either by asking direct questions or by asking hidden questions (see chapter 2) and the nurse should try to be aware of hidden messages when conveying personally-threatening information.

Reluctance to carry out self-care

The second circumstance in which a patient may reject information is where the information relates to self-care instructions which the patient believes are ineffective, personally unacceptable, unpleasant or not worth pursuing. For example, a bronchitic patient may not wish to give up smoking despite being told that his condition is directly linked to this.

The extent to which patients reject information is difficult to assess. The only related data comes from studies examining whether patients comply with instructions, although failure to comply with instructions may be caused by one or more of three things: failing to understand the instructions, failing to remember the instructions or failing to accept the instructions.

Studies on patient compliance (for reviews see Baekeland and Lundwell, 1975; Dunbar and Agras, 1980; Ley, 1979) show that compliance with, for instance, advice on taking drugs, on dieting and on attending antenatal classes is often very low. Research on compliance with drug-taking instructions shows that non-compliance is generally unaffected by the type of drug involved (Ley, 1982) and in some studies as many as 50 per cent of patients are not complying with advice.

It is important to recognise that only some patients will choose not to follow advice. Many patients believe that the nurse or doctor 'knows best' and will follow advice even if it seems silly to to so. In fact, if such highly compliant patients misunderstand or misremember instructions they can do things which are quite dangerous. One should certainly question whether it is beneficial for patients to behave in a way in which they relinquish all sense of self-determination in health care to 'the experts'. A perception of competence or control is important (see chapters 1 and 9) and it is worth noting that a tendency not to comply with instructions unless convinced may be psychologically healthy.

Aiding compliance

There are several factors which affect whether a patient thinks advice is worth following. These factors will be described under the following headings: (a) the patient's relationship with the information-giver, (b) the credibility of the information-giver, (c) presenting a balanced argument, (d) reasons for treatment, (e) self-disclosure by the patient, (f) fear, (g) the patient's medical understanding, and (h) practical considerations.

The relationship with the information-giver

Patients are more likely to be convinced by an argument if they like the person who is putting it forward. In a review of 35 studies, Baekeland and Lundwall (1975) found that, in all cases, compliance was better where staff had good relationships with their patients. A good therapeutic relationship (see chapter 2) is therefore an important part of persuading patients to follow advice.

The credibility of the information-giver

A credible person is someone who is perceived to be trustworthy and have an expert knowledge. Patients are more likely to follow advice given by someone who appears credible than someone who does not (Hovland and Weiss, 1951). Although nurses and doctors are often perceived as credible, it is important for them to maintain their credibility by being honest. Bluffing is almost always found out by patients, and leads to the conclusion that the professional is untrustworthy. Credibility will also be lost if information is withheld and the patient discovers this later.

Research shows that physically attractive communicators are perceived to be more credible (Mills and Aronson, 1965), as are people who have had similar experiences to the patient or client (Berscheid, 1966). Self-help groups, where individuals with similar problems meet, are often effective in helping people to accept information or comply with instructions, because the other group members are preceived as having credibility.

Presenting a balanced argument

Suppose the nurse wants to persuade a mother to breast feed her baby. Should she present only the positive reasons for breast-feeding (e.g. better immunological protection for the baby) or should she present both the positive reasons for, and also the negative consequences of, breast-feeding (e.g. that it is more time-consuming)?

In general, the two-sided argument works better, particularly if the person appears to be questioning what is suggested, or if relatives disagree with the advice. The two-sided argument makes the communicator appear more credible than does the one-sided argument, as it appears that she has a more complete picture of the problem (Hovland, Lumsdaine and Sheffield, 1949).

There are, however, occasions when the one-sided argument is more effective. If the patient is inclined to do what is proposed it is only necessary to provide one side of the information. Also, if the client is likely to be confused by trying to understand several opposing arguments at the same time it is better to give only one side of the argument.

Giving reasons for treatment

Many forms of treatment or self-care have unwanted side-effects. Some drugs induce drowsiness, others cause nausea. Dieting leads to hunger, while exercise is time-consuming and requires effort.

However, the negative side-effects of treatment should always be discussed. It can be counter-productive for patients suddenly to discover these side-effects as they may think that something is going wrong with their treatment. If side-effects are very rare, the nurse has to use her discretion as to whether or not to discuss them, as the patient may worry unnecessarily or imagine problems when they are not present. In general, however, patients should be told about possible side-effects, because only by knowing about them do they have the necessary information to make an informed choice.

To be persuasive, it is necessary to argue that it is worth putting up with the negative effects of treatment or self-care. One way to achieve this is to give reasons for the treatment. Instructions for treatment should never be given without reasons. The patient must also know how the self-care procedure achieves its effect, how long it is likely to take and what is likely to happen in the interim.

It is important to accept that there may be a rational reason for the patient not following the carer's advice, as he may value different things in life from the carer. For example, the patient may decide to continue smoking even though he knows it might kill him because he believes that life is not worth living without smoking. The patient makes a free choice as to whether the professional's advice is worth following.

Cameron and Gregor (1987) say, in their 'health belief' model, that the patient weighs up the costs and benefits of complying with instructions.

Self-disclosure

One reason why people are sometimes reluctant to follow advice is that, by following advice, they feel they are relinquishing their sense of self-determination and control. Indeed, if one is trying to convince someone of something, the listener is more likely to be convinced if he thinks it is his idea rather than someone else's. In the example of Mrs Rogers and the nurse given above, the nurse let Mrs Rogers decide that her smoking might have affected her baby, and the nurse also let Mrs Rogers decide on her own to give up smoking: she did not order Mrs Rogers to give up smoking.

Langer (1983) suggests that when patients describe their problems and follow advice they expose themselves to a feeling of loss of control. Langer suggests that one way round this feeling of loss is for the nurse or communicator to engage in *reciprocal self-disclosure*. That is, the nurse talks about herself and her own problems as a way of making the patient feel more in control of the situation. Interestingly, reciprocal self-disclosure is the normal pattern of interaction between people: usually if one person discloses a secret, the other feels obliged to reciprocate with a secret of his own. There is some evidence in support of Langer's hypothesis (Langer, Rodin, Beck Weinman and Spitzer, 1979).

The use of self-disclosure as a way of improving a patient's sense of control can be most usefully employed where the interaction between patient and nurse occurs over a period of time. Reciprocal self-disclosure is a potentially useful tool, particularly where a nurse suspects that a patient is reacting negatively to perceived loss of control. However, the nurse should limit the amount of self-disclosure lest the patient think that the nurse is more concerned about herself than about the patient.

Fear

In telling the patient the purpose of a self-care procedure, it is possible to present a very frightening picture of what will happen if he does not comply. The ethics of producing such frightening scenarios should be considered. The research in this area (Dabbs and Leventhal, 1966; Janis and Feshbach, 1953) suggests that making a person afraid is effective only if that person has adequate coping strategies for dealing with the feared outcome. Frightening people about something which they can avoid only with difficulty is not a good idea. Under such circumstances, people may avoid fear by simply not listening to what they are told. In the example of Dr J and Mrs Ellis, Dr J tried using the 'sledgehammer' technique of frightening Mrs Ellis into doing the right thing. Mrs Ellis could not easily give up smoking, so this led to a rejection of both Dr J and his advice.

A useful rule to follow is to induce only low levels of fear. If a point of view is stresed too forcefully, more resistance than agreement may ensue. Tales about horrible deaths which happen to people who do not do what they are told not only appear unethical but are often also counter-productive: they can lead to the 'sod you' effect (see above).

The patient's medical understanding

Patients may not follow self-care advice because it conflicts with their own understanding of medical matters. For example, some patients do not like taking pills because they feel they ought to be able to cope on their own, and some have highly inaccurate views about the cause and treatment of an illness (Ley and Spelman, 1967).

People may feel that they really know about the cause of their illness whereas doctors and nurses have got it all wrong. When patients question the authority of medical and nursing staff, there is no point in taking an authoritarian approach. It is unproductive for the carer to say, 'I have been in this job for 20 years and I know what is best for you'. Patients who question advice—and wrong advice can be given—will only be convinced by rational argument. Under these circumstances, a good course of action is for the carer to give more medical details to the patient and, as suggested earlier, to present both sides of the argument.

The nurse may give advice opposite to that being given by the patient's relatives. If she suspects that the patient perhaps (or his carer) is being subjected to 'counter-propaganda', she should try to find out the basis of this and counter it with rational argument. The patient should be given a reason to support the counter-propaganda– but a better reason to support what the nurse suggests.

It is often very difficult to support a patient against outside influence when the patient is at home, because the nurse has only occasional contact with the patient, whereas relatives may have constant contact. Some battles cannot be won despite the nurse's best efforts.

● A young Chinese woman who had two young children was in the remission stage of a cancer, with a good prognosis. However, the woman's mother was convinced that cancer was contagious. She insisted that the mother was kept away from her own children and also that she should eat in a separate room. Despite the nursing staff contacting a spokesman from the Chinese legation to try to explain the situation to the grandmother, the problem was never satisfactorily resolved.

Practical considerations

Several practical factors can prevent patients following advice. Research (Dunbar and Agras, 1980) shows that inconvenient, complex regimens of self-care are followed less often than simple ones. One way of reducing the inconvenience of care is through careful management of the patient's time.

● An antenatal clinic in Hospital A is run in the following way. All expectant mothers arrive at 2 p.m., are given dressing-gowns and are asked to wait. Some expectant mothers have to wait two or three hours before they are dealt with. Not surprisingly, attendance is lower than in Hospital B where appointments are made on an individual basis.

Long waiting times have been shown to be associated with missed appointments, and block bookings of patients (where all patients arrive at the same time) are worse in this respect than individually booked appointments (Dunbar and Agras, 1980).

Because doctors and nurses often see things from their own point of view (e.g. the smooth running of a hospital or clinic or the patient's recovery) they often fail to see things from the patient's point of view (e.g. the smooth running of a home or career). Moores and Thompson (1986) found that more than half of the hospital patients they questioned thought that nurses had routine duties to follow and patients had somehow to fit in with these duties. Cameron and Gregor (1987) distinguish the patient's view of a suggested regimen, and how it affects the patient's life, from the nurse's view of a suggested regimen and how it affects the patient's health. A skilful nurse will take the trouble to find out how a treatment schedule affects the patient's life.

In summary, a nurse should try to make it easy, not difficult, for the patient to follow self-care instructions. She should try to find out about the practical, day-to-day concerns which affect the patient's self-care and, if a patient does not follow advice, the nurse should ask why. Good advice starts from understanding the patient's viewpoint.

SUMMARY

This chapter covers the role of the nurse as a giver of information. Nurses play a crucial role in providing patients with information, yet research shows that patients are often dissatisfied with the information they receive, which can be harmful to good health care.

Covered in this chapter are:

1. How to give information in ways which help people *understand* what is being said

2. How to give information in ways which help people *remember* what is being said

3. How to give information in ways which help people *accept* what is being said

Good communication between nurse and patient is individualised. In order to individualise the information she gives, the nurse must first assess the patient in terms of his psychological state, preferred style of communication and communication needs. Skilful information-giving starts from skilful questioning: an efficient communicator makes a thorough assessment before providing information.

References

Baekeland F and Lundwall L (1975) Dropping out of treatment: a critical review. *Psychological Bulletin*, **82**: 738–783.
Berscheid E (1966) Opinion change and communicator–communicatee similarity and dissimilarity. *Journal of Personality and Social Psychology*, **4**: 670–680.
Boyle C M (1970) Differences between doctor's and patient's interpretations of some common medical terms. *British Medical Journal*, **ii**: 286–289.
Cameron K and Gregor F (1987) Chronic illness and compliance. *Journal of Advanced Nursing*, **12**: 671–676.
Cartwright A (1964) *Human Relations and Hospital Care*. London: Routledge and Kegan Paul.
Crotty M (1985) Communication between nurses and their patients. *Nurse Education Today*, **5**: 130–134.
Dabbs J M and Leventhal H (1966) Effects of varying the recommendations in fear arousing communication. *Journal of Personality and Social Psychology*, **4**: 525–531.

Dunbar J M and Agras W S (1980) Compliance with medical instructions. In: *The Comprehensive Handbook of Behavioral Medicine*, eds. Ferguson J M and Taylor C B, vol. 3, pp. 115–145. Lancaster: M T P Press.

Engstrom B (1984) The patient's need for information during hospital stay. *International Journal of Nursing Studies*, **21**: 113–130.

French K (1981) Methodological considerations in hospital patient opinion surveys. *International Journal of Nursing Studies*, **18**: 7–32.

Hovland C I, Lumsdaine A A and Sheffield F D (1949) *Experiments on Mass Communication*, Princeton, New Jersey: Princeton University Press.

Hovland C I and Weiss W (1951) The influence of source credibility on communication effectiveness. *Public Opinion Quarterly*, **15**: 635–650.

Humphreys M S and Revelle W (1984) Personality, motivation and performance: a theory of the relationship between individual differences and information processing. *Psychological Review*, **91**: 153–184.

Inguanzo J M and Harju M (1985) Consumer satisfaction with hospitalization. *Hospitals*, **59(9)**: 81–83.

Janis I L and Feshbach S (1953) Effects of fear-arousing communications. *Journal of Abnormal and Social Psychology*, **48**: 78–92.

Langer E J (1983) *The Psychology of Control*. Beverley Hills, California: Sage.

Langer E J, Rodin J, Beck P, Weinman C and Spitzer L (1979) Environmental determinants of memory improvement in late adulthood. *Journal of Personality and Social Psychology*, **37**: 2003–2013.

Ley P (1979) The psychology of compliance. In: *Research in Psychology and Medicine*, Chourne D J, Gruneberg M M and Eiser J R, eds. vol. **2**, pp.187–202. London: Academic Press.

Ley P (1982) Satisfaction, compliance and communication. *British Journal of Clinical Psychology*, **21**: 241–254.

Ley P and Spelman M S (1965) Communications in an out-patient setting. *British Journal of Social and Clinical Psychology*, **4**: 114–116.

Ley P and Spelman M S (1967) *Communicating with the Patient*. London: Staples Press.

McGhee A (1961) *The Patient's Attitude to Nursing Care*. Edinburgh: Churchill Livingstone.

MacStravic R S (1986) Therapeutic pampering. *Hospital and Health Services Administration*, **31**: 59–69.

Mills J and Aronson E (1965) Opinion change as a function of the communicator's attractiveness and desire to influence. *Journal of Personality and Social Psychology*, **1**: 173–177.

Moores B and Thompson A G H (1986) What 1357 hospital inpatients think about aspects of their stay in British acute hospitals. *Journal of Advanced Nursing*, **11**: 86–102.

Riley C S (1966) Patients' understanding of doctors' instructions. *Medical Care*, **4**: 34–37.

4
Individual Differences

Every person is in certain respects (a) like all other people, (b) like some other people, (c) like no other person (adapted from Kluckhohn and Murray, 1953, p.53). This means that in some respects patients are the same and can be cared for in the same way; in some respects patients are like some people but different from others and require care which is appropriate to their particular type; and in other respects each patient is unique and requires a unique form of care. This chapter provides information about ways in which different types of people require different forms of management. It is divided into three main sections.

1. Personality: the psychological differences between people which have been investigated through research, and the implications of those differences for nursing practice.

2. Common-sense ways of understanding personality and the way in which people make judgments about others.

3. Differences between the sexes and in particular in sexual behaviour.

The aims of this chapter are (a) to increase awareness of the ways in which people differ and how to care for people depending on their different characteristics; (b) to help nurses to be good and careful judges of personality; (c) to encourage a way of assessing people which avoids approval or disapproval of the way in which they live.

PERSONALITY FROM A PSYCHOLOGICAL PERSPECTIVE

What is personality?

Whatever a person does, his behaviour results from a combination of two factors:

- internal or 'person' characteristics;
- external or situational characteristics.

This idea is expressed diagramatically in figure 4.1.

Personality is one of the 'person' characteristics; other 'person' characteristics include memory and mood state. Personality, like other 'person' characteristics, cannot be seen. Instead, personality is inferred from behaviour.

Personality and situation do not necessarily contribute equally to behaviour. Sometimes the situation is the more important factor and at other times, personality.

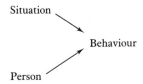

Fig. 4.1 Determinants of behaviour

For example, when a student sits down to listen to a lecture, it is the situation rather than his personality which is responsible for the behaviour of sitting. It will be obvious that personality cannot be inferred from behaviour which is caused by the situation but only from that which is caused by personality.

In general, when people behave in the same way in a particular situation the situation is the cause of behaviour (consider the example of sitting in a lecture theatre). However, if people behave in different ways in the same situation personality may be responsible for this difference. If one student is constantly standing up and telling jokes to the rest of the class, then we are likely to infer that there is something unusual about that student's personality.

In some respects, differences in behaviour between people are consistently different across different situations. For example, one person may tell jokes in all kinds of circumstances whereas another may never tell jokes. This form of consistency exhibited by a person allows behaviour to be predicted from one situation to another, and forms the basis for the study of personality. Personality for an individual is defined as that which causes behaviour to be consistent in different situations.

If a patient is aggressive on the ward as well as at home, the patient could be described as having an aggressive personality. However, if the patient was aggressive only on the ward, then it would not be true to say that the patient had an aggressive personality because the patient's behaviour fails to be consistent across different situations. To take another example, consider a patient who is grumpy and irritable when ill but charming when well. The patient may appear to be a grumpy person to the nursing staff, but he has not got an irritable personality. His grumpiness is a reponse to a particular situation: that of being ill.

This section has two aims. The first is to alert the nurse to the variety of ways in which people differ. Four of the many types of personality theory will be described.

1. Theories involving different sorts of needs or goals
2. Theories involving different levels of intellectual ability
3. Theories involving different sorts of trait.
4. Reversal theory

The second aim of this section is to show how people with different personalities may need different forms of care.

Need theories of personality

It is an accepted fact that people have needs, goals or motives for which they strive. Murray (1938) produced a list of some 30 needs, a list which he developed intuitively on the basis of hours of counselling interviews. Murray's list includes the need for achievement, the need for affiliation and the need for power. In their activities for living, Roper et al (1980) list 12 needs which they feel are important to nursing. These needs are maintaining a safe environment, communicating, breathing, eating and drinking, eliminating, personal cleansing and dressing, controlling body temperature, mobilising, working and playing, expressing sexuality, sleeping and dying. They are sometimes used as the basis of an assessment tool. Henderson (1966) lists 14 needs which are similar to Roper's but with the addition of the need to worship. Notice that some of these needs are physical needs (e.g. eating, breathing and eliminating) whereas others are psychological needs (e.g. communicating, playing and worshipping). The psychological needs are those relevant for psychological care of the patient.

It is important to realise that these lists of needs are arbitrary. There is no scientific basis for the particular needs listed by Murray, Roper or Henderson. All these lists were developed in a practical context to satisfy a practical need. They should not be treated as a definitive statement of the needs of a patient, but as a starting point for assessment.

There are other needs not mentioned in these lists. For example, learned helplessness theory, discussed in chapter 1, is based on the assumption that people have a need for control or self-determination; that is, a need to feel that they can control themselves and their environment (White, 1959). The need for control is listed neither by Roper nor by Murray yet is important from the point of view of psychological care. Another important need is the need for information (see chapter 2). There are many other needs which psychologists believe are important to psychological well-being but which do not form part of traditional lists. These include the need for self-esteem and the need to understand the meaning of one's life, the latter often becoming important to people who are dying.

There is an almost limitless number of goals for which an individual can strive and different people strive for different ones. Any list of needs is best thought of as being composed of common categories of need. When assessing the patient, the nurse should try to find out precisely what needs he has within each category as well as find out about needs which do not fall into any of these common categories.

● A young man was admitted to Dorset ward. He arrived wearing a black leather jacket with metal studs attached. On the ward he was extremely withdrawn and quiet. One of the nurses discovered that the patient had a strong need to have a 'macho' image and was having difficulty coping with the loss of his normal perception of himself. He could be helped by the nurse making positive comparisons with people who had been in hospital and whom the patient would admire, e.g. racing drivers or motor-bike riders, thereby showing that it was 'normal' for people like himself to be hospitalised. Alternatively, the nurse could move the man's bed so he could be near others like himself.

Not only do people have different goals but they also strive for those goals with different levels of intensity. For example, the strength of the need to control the environment varies between people. Those who have a high need for control but find themselves to be helpless find their circumstances to be more unpleasant than those who have only a weak need for control. In such situations the former are more likely to have suicidal thoughts (Burger, 1984).

The need for achievement (i.e. the need to reach excellence) has been the focus for one theory of personality (Atkinson and Birch, 1978). Some people have a strong need to achieve, others only have a weak one. Some nursing students are more strongly motivated than others to pass their exams and as a result revise more. People with strong motives are more likely to feel depressed when their goals are not reached than are people with weak motives. Those with a strong need for achievement try harder to reach excellence, but are also more prone to be upset if they are prevented from achieving their goals.

● On admission, Mr McFarlane behaved like a model patient and cooperated well with the nursing staff. However, towards the end of his stay, he became rather demanding and constantly requested the telephone trolley to be brought to his bed. It transpired that Mr McFarlane wanted to continue working while still in hospital.

Research on achievement motivation (Atkinson and Birch, 1978) shows that the achievement goal is made up of two components: the need for success and the need to avoid failure. These two needs can conflict with each other. To succeed at a task it is necessary to have a go at the task but, to avoid failure, all that may be necessary is to avoid having a go. For example, a patient who is trying to walk may have a conflict between attempting to walk, an action which may be successful, and putting off trying to walk, thereby avoiding failure. For some people the need for success is greater than the need to avoid failure, whereas for others the need to avoid failure is more important than the need for success, and in a given situation these two types will behave differently.

People who have a high need for success but a low fear of failure need a challenge. They work hardest when there is a moderate chance of failure, but work less hard when they are being successful. Patients with a high for need for success are comparatively easy to rehabilitate because they rise to the challenge of their limitations.

People who have a high fear of failure and a low need for success, on the other hand, tend to give up when there is a moderate chance of failure but work hardest when there is a good chance of success. Such patients can be more difficult to rehabilitate, particularly if there is the possibility of the patient failing at what he is doing.

We all need some encouragement; we all have a need to feel that we are doing well. However, some patients—and some nurses—need more encouragement than others. Patients who are in particular need of encouragement consist of those who are high in fear of failure and those who experience goal conflict between wanting and not wanting to do a particular task.

High fear of failure

How can one give encouragement to people who think they are going to fail, individuals who are characterised by high levels of anxiety? The best way to approach the problem is in terms of attributions (see chapter 1) which are the perceived causes for an event. Internal attributions are made when the cause of an event is believed to be some characteristic of the person; external attributions are made when the cause of an event is thought to be an aspect of the situation, e.g. other people. Long-term attributions are made when the cause is unlikely to change, and short-term attributions when the cause is of only a temporary nature.

People high in the need to avoid failure tend to explain their own failures in terms of internal and long-term characteristics (Weiner, 1980). For example, a student nurse who has just failed an assignment may think that this failure is caused by her being 'too stupid', a personality characteristic which is internal (a characteristic of the student) and also long term (i.e. unlikely to change). Therefore, the nurse expects to fail future exams and may even consider giving up nursing. A patient who is having difficulty walking may say that she is never going to be able to walk because 'she hasn't got it in her'.

The secret of giving encouragement to a patient who fears failure is to find out why he thinks he is not doing well or is likely to fail. Having ascertained the patient's attributions, the nurse should then give, and try to convince the patient of, an alternative, more positive, attribution, i.e. either an external or a short-term explanation for failure. For example, the student nurse could be told that her failure was a matter of luck because she 'wasn't asked the questions she was expecting' (i.e. an external attribution), or that it was just an 'off day' (i.e. a short-term one). The patient could be told that her difficulty with walking was only occurring because she was 'trying too soon' (a short-term cause). Encouraging people involves giving them a positive interpretation of what has happened in the past and not just relying on telling them that they are going to do well in the future. To encourage, the nurse needs to find out what the patient thinks is causing the problem, i.e. she must make a psychological assessment of the patient as well as a physical one.

To some extent it does not matter what really causes one to succeed or fail; it is what one believes that is important. Generally, people try harder and get more out of their work if they can take pride in their success by attributing success to themselves (i.e. 'I passed the examination because I am so brilliant'), and they protect themselves from failure by blaming other things or people.

When a patient with a high fear of failure is being rehabilitated he should be given plenty of encouragement and should be set easy goals to accomplish, so that he is protected from the experience of failure. If a patient appears to be afraid of failing in a task (for example, walking to the bathroom) he should be told how well he is doing, and the task should be divided into easily accomplished sub-tasks (for example, sitting on bed, then standing next to bed, next walking with stick or frame etc.).

It is useful to distinguish 'nursing goals' from 'patient-centred goals.' The nursing goal may be for the patient to walk, but the patient may have other more limited goals, such as sitting in a chair. It is better to take things in easy stages and concentrate on the patient's own goals rather than focus the patient's attention exclusively on the nurse's goal. There is no point in talking about the lovely view from the top of a mountain when someone has a broken leg and is worrying about reaching the lavatory.

Goal conflict

There is another side to encouragement. The need for success and the need to avoid failure sometimes conflict with each other, and a patient may experience this conflict by both wanting and not wanting to try to reach his goal. Sometimes a patient who experiences a conflict between needs can be recognised through 'channel disparity' in which the verbal and non-verbal messages fail to mesh (see chapter 2). For example, if a nurse asks the patient if he would like to get up and the patient smiles and says,

'No', the nurse might infer that part of the patient is saying 'No' and part is saying 'Yes'. Under these circumstances, encouragement can be given by being more directive and, in effect, telling the patient what to do. When the patient experiences a conflict between goals, he will react best if the nurse gives a one-sided argument supporting the goal which the nurse wishes to endorse. The goal conflict patient is already half way to success: he just needs pushing in the right direction.

Patients experiencing goal conflict can be encouraged with statements like, 'Come on, Mr Smith, you're ready to get up now and I am sure you can do it'. Patients experiencing goal conflict should be managed differently from patients who are simply greatly afraid of failure. Patients need different types of encouragement depending on their personality.

Hierarchical organisation of goals

One of the weaknesses of presenting goals in list-form is that it fails to draw attention to the fact that goals are interrelated. Goals are arranged hierarchically. Those lower down in the hierarchy are the 'means' to the 'ends', the 'end' being a goal towards the top of the hierarchy (Hyland, 1987).

Let us use the typical goals of a nurse as an example. A nurse has a goal to carry out a particular procedure, for example, giving an injection. By carrying out the procedure well (or more specifically, by believing she carries it out well), she satisfies her need to see herself as a good, caring nurse. Knowledge that she is a caring nurse satisfies her need for self-determination (Deci and Ryan, 1985), which in turn helps to satisfy her need for self-esteem. These needs can be laid out as in figure 4.2, some additional needs also being added.

Figure 4.2 shows that the need for self-esteem is satisfied by success in the lower level goals. Of course, one could be successful at any one of a number of possible goals, but success in something is needed for positive self-esteem.

This organisation of goals has a very important implication for nursing: failure to achieve some apparently trivial goal may have serious consequences for a patient's high-level goals. For example, an elderly female patient may find herself unable to look after her husband as well as she used to (the husband being perfectly capable of

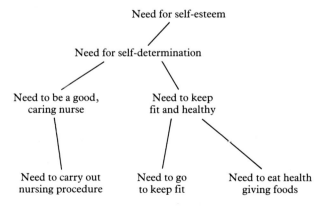

Fig. 4.2 A causal hierarchy of goals

looking after himself). She may find this inability threatening to her self-esteem and self-determination, both needs having been satisfied in the past by her ability to look after her spouse. What is a trivial goal to the nurse may be a very important goal to the patient.

It is very important for the nurse to think about goals as being interrelated and the failure to satisfy any one goal as having implications for other goals. For example, Roper lists 'elimination' in her activities for living. Many people who suffer from incontinence find that 'accidents' are socially distressing and lead to lack of dignity; it is the loss of self-esteem which matters to them, not the accident. A nurse is much better able to advise a patient if she is aware of the patient's social distress from such a physical problem.

There is another aspect to the interrelationship of goals. It is that attaining one goal can get in the way of attaining other goals. For example, it may be difficult (though by no means impossible) to be a full-time nurse and an effective mother. This depends, of course, on what one means by 'being an effective mother' as people have different goals of motherhood. A nurse should also try to be aware of the conflicts which can be experienced in trying to achieve a number of sometimes incompatible goals. Conflict between goals is not always inevitable, and changes can be made which might remove conflict. For instance, the conflict between the roles of nurse and mother can be alleviated by changing the social environment e.g. by providing creches in hospitals.

Intellectual ability: theories of intelligence

People appear to differ in terms of something which we call 'intelligence', and this level of 'intelligence' can be quantified by using an intelligence quotient (or IQ) test. However, the commonly-accepted view of intelligence is not entirely correct, and the purpose of this section is to disourage nurses from classifying people simply as 'bright' or 'stupid'.

The scientific study of intelligence began in the early 1900s when Charles Spearman gave tests for various sorts of mental ability to children (Spearman, 1927). Spearman found that the difference sorts of test seemed to correlate with each other (see below) and he therefore assumed that there was some common, underlying, 'general factor' of intelligence which was reflected in all the different tests. Spearman called this general factor 'g', but recognised that there were other specific types of intelligence which were independent of 'g'. He called these specific types of intelligence 's'. An IQ score is a measure of general intelligence, and is arrived at by averaging the scores from a number of different specific tests.

Spearman believed that some of the different types of intelligence were closely related to each other, i.e. showed a strong correlation. *Correlation* is a statistical procedure for examining the relationship between two *variables*, a variable simply being something which varies. A person's height and weight are both variables. In general, tall people tend to be heavier than short people which, from a statistical point of view, means that height and weight are correlated. Of course, some short people are very heavy and there are some tall people who are light. The correlation between height and weight simply means that there is a tendency for tall people to be heavy. The strength of this tendency can be expressed numerically by the use of a number called a *correlation coefficient*.

Subsequent research (see Shackleton and Fletcher, 1984) established that there were at least four specific types of intelligence: verbal, arithmetical, spatial and mechanical. Some researchers, however, argue that there are many more types of specific intelligence and some believe that the different sorts of specific intelligence are, in fact, so poorly related with each other (i.e. they have such low correlations) that it is a mistake to talk about general intelligence (in the singular), and one should properly speak of specific intelligences (in the plural).

Whatever the strengths of the arguments between these different researchers, it is clear that specific intelligences do exist, even if there is also a general factor. The moral of this story is that some people are intelligent in one way, but not so bright in another. Just because a person has poor verbal ability there is no reason to write him off as being 'unintelligent': he may be very good at arithmetic. And because someone is good at one type of mental activity does not mean that he is going to be good at all types.

From the point of view of nursing, research into intelligence shows that judgments about a person's general intelligence may not be the most useful personality dimension from the point of view of patient management. It is far better to find out about a patient's specific strengths and weaknesses than to use a general category of intelligence to assess him.

Trait theories of personality

A *trait* is a style of behaviour in a person which is consistent across different situations. In psychology, there are many theories which focus on different styles of behaviour. Eysenck's theory of personality (Eysenck, 1952) is a well known theory which is based on two traits, *extroversion–introversion*, and *neurotisicm–stability*.

The terms 'extrovert' and 'introvert' are labels for traits which tend to go together. An extrovert is sociable, impulsive, active, lively and excitable. An introvert, on the other hand, is quiet, introspective, avoids excitement, likes a well-ordered life and is reliable. Extroversion–introversion represents a dimension or continuum. According to Eysenck everyone can be located on this continuum, each person having a place on the line below.

Introversion . . . . Extroversion

In fact, the majority of people fall somewhere in the middle of the line so they are neither strongly extrovert nor strongly introvert. These 'in-between' people are called 'ambiverts'. The terms 'introvert' and 'extrovert' are most usefully applied to a much smaller number of people who are at either end of the line.

Eysenck suggests that there is a biological basis for the difference between extroverts and introverts. He believes that extroverts have relatively weak cortical activity, that is the cells in the cortex (the part of the brain which is responsible for thought) are relatively inactive. In order to achieve a higher level of cortical activity, which is the preferred level, extroverts seek stimulation. Introverts, on the other hand, have high levels of cortical activity but prefer a lower level. Consequently, introverts try to reduce cortical activity by avoiding stimulation. Thus, extroverts are stimulus-seekers and introverts are stimulus-avoiders.

Research has shown that introverts and extroverts (as measured by a personality questionnaire) do prefer to be in different situations and perform differently under different conditions. Extroverts prefer, and work better under, conditions where there is plenty of activity. Introverts, however, perform better on tasks where there is a relatively low level of stimulation. For example, radar operators who spend much of their time looking at a screen waiting for a 'blip' to show are often introverts rather than extroverts. Extroverted nurses will become bored with repetitive tasks with which introverts cope well. However, introverts will find stressful those situations which extroverts find exciting.

Introverts and extroverts differ in terms of their tolerance of sensory deprivation. Consider what it must be like to break several limbs and be encased in plaster in hospital. The extrovert will find the experience much more aversive than the introvert. Under such circumstances, the experience can be made less unpleasant for the extrovert by placing him in a busy, noisy ward. Introverts, on the other hand, are likely to prefer less busy ward environments.

Eysenck also suggests a second personality dimension, neuroticism–stability which, like extroversion–introversion, he suggests has a biological basis. He hypothesises that neurotic people have highly reactive sympathetic nervous systems. The sympathetic nervous system comprises involuntary nerves which prepare the body for 'fight or flight' under situations of stress. The sympathetic nervous system, for example, increases a person's heart rate when he has a sudden surprise. In some people, the sympathetic nervous system is particularly reactive to stressful events. The consequence of this is that some people, those at the neurotic end of the continuum shown below, are more likely to react strongly to worries and anxieties.

Neurotic . . . . Stable

The important thing to realise about the neurotic personality is that this individual reacts badly only under conditions of stress, as, under conditions of calm and relaxation, the sympathetic nervous system is not active. In such circumstances those with a neurotic tendency are more likely to be upset, both psychologically, than their more stable counterparts.

Evidence that neurotic people tend to react badly to illness come from studies (reviewed in Mathew and Ridgeway, 1981) showing that people classified as neurotic on Eysenck's personality questionnaire report more pain, have longer hospital stays and have more respiratory complications following surgery. This poor reaction may be because certain hormones produced during periods of stress inhibit recovery (see chapter 7) and people with highly reactive sympathetic nervous systems will produce more of these stress hormones.

It was shown in chapter 2 that people sometimes do not remember what they are told because they are too anxious or aroused. This tendency to forget due to over-arousal is more likely with a neurotic personality, and with these patients the nurse needs to take special care to communicate under conditions of calm and relaxation and not, for example, on a busy ward round.

Reversal theory

All the theories of personality described above assume that the personality contribution to behaviour is constant over time. For example, an extrovert always tends to be an extrovert. Reversal theory (Apter, 1984), on the other hand, suggests that the personality component changes over time. According to this approach, people switch between different 'modes' and there are different styles of experiencing and behaving associated with each mode.

The two modes, forming a pair, which have received most research attention are the *telic* and *paratelic*. Someone in the telic mode is goal-oriented, serious, tends to plan ahead and prefers low levels of arousal. Someone in the paratelic mode is not goal-oriented, is playful, does not plan ahead and prefers high levels of arousal. The telic mode is the mode associated with working, the paratelic mode that associated with play. Thus, people switch between a working, or telic, mode of behaviour and playful, or paratelic, mode.

Apter suggests that when someone is in the telic mode, low arousal is experienced as relaxation and high arousal as anxiety. However, when in the paratelic mode, low arousal is experienced as boredom and high arousal as excitement.

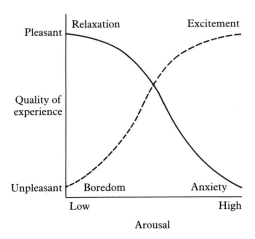

Fig. 4.3 Diagram illustrating telic (——) and paratelic (– – –) modes

The implication of this theory for nursing is that a person's behaviour is likely to change depending on which mode he is in. For example, a patient may become very disruptive when in the paratelic state because the arousal which results from being disruptive is experienced as excitement. However, if the patient can be made to focus on certain goals, i.e. to shift into the telic mode, the disruptive behaviour should stop, as the high arousal is then experienced as anxiety. Thus, one way of dealing with disruptive behaviour is to talk to the patient in a way which encourages the patient to plan ahead.

● Les Johnson was admitted to the casualty department in a highly disruptive state. He shouted at anyone who was passing and obviously enjoyed upsetting people in the waiting area. When a nurse started talking to Les about his problem he became much more amenable and quietened down. As a result of the nurse's action Les had shifted from being in the paratelic to the telic state.

Reversal theory suggests that people naturally switch between states. People like to be serious and work at times and at other times like to play and enjoy themselves. Some people like to have fun more often than others but, even so, everyone at some time shifts between the telic and paratelic modes. It is, therefore, important for nurses to realise that people do have the need to shift into an excitement-seeking mode of behaivour.

Apter (1984) suggests that although all people switch between modes some people tend to be more often in the telic mode, i.e. *telic dominant*, whereas others tend to be more often in the paratelic mode, i.e. *paratelic dominant*. People tend to become more telic dominant as they grow older, so young adults and teenagers are more likely to be paratelic dominant. It is particularly useful, for young, long-stay patients, to have a legitimate way of (occasionally) becoming excited during what can otherwise be a very boring sojourn in hosptial.

Summary and overview of section on personality

The purpose of this section has been to show the variety of ways in which people differ as expressed through psychological theories of personality and to show how different types of patient require different forms of care.

Four kinds of theory were discussed in this section.

1. *Need theories* show how people differ in terms of the goals they have, the intensity with which they seek those goals, and the hierarchical organisation of those goals. Need theories help a nurse to understand patients, to give patients encouragement and to be aware of possible conflicts between goals.

2. *Theories of intelligence* show how people differ in terms of intellectual ability. There are many different types of intellectual ability and a nurse should not assume that just because someone is weak in one type of ability he is not strong in some other area.

3. *Trait theories* show that people differ in terms of behavioural traits. The traits of extroversion–introversion and neuroticism–stability form part of Eysenck's theory. Extroverts and introverts differ in terms of their preferred level of stimulation, and neurotics have a greater autonomic response to stressful events than more stable people.

4. *Reversal theory* suggests that people reverse between modes and that people behave and experience things differently in different modes. The arousal-seeking telic mode and the arousal-avoiding paratelic mode were discussed, together with their implications for nursing with regard to disruptive behaviour and long-term care.

In summary, people are different in many different ways. When assessing the psychological characteristics of a patient, it is clearly not possible to give out personality questionnaires but it is useful to keep in mind the many ways in which psychologists have found people differ.

JUDGING OTHER PEOPLE

Although psychologists have studied personality for over a century, one does not need to be a psychologist to make an assessment of another's personality. People frequently make judgments about personality and are often quite confident about their ability to 'know what others are really like'. Psychologists have also studied how the layman assesses personality, and some of the confidence people have when judging others has been shown to be unfounded. This section examines the psychology of judging other people.

Personal constructs

The most common concept used when judging another person is that of a trait. In the English language there are over 3 000 trait words, so there are a variety of traits which can be used. Any single person, however, only uses a relatively small number of trait words when describing others. The particular trait words used by a person when judging another constitutes that person's own theory of personality, their *implicit personality theory*.

Repertory grid test

How can a person's implicit personality theory by uncovered? A technique called the repertory grid test allows this to be done and is described below (see Bannister and Fransella, 1971, for more detail).

1. The subject writes down a list of about 10 people known to him.

2. He then takes three people at random from the list and thinks of a way in which two are similar and one different. For example, two of the people may be easy to get on with and the other not so easy to get on with. This can be written as:

     Easy to get on with . . . . Not easy to get on with

   This continuum is called a *construct*.

3. Another three people are then selected from the list and the same procedure followed to produce another construct. For example, the new construct might be:

     Placid . . . . Irritable

4. This should be continued until no new constructs can be produced. This final list of constructs or dimensions is that which the subject commonly uses for judging people.

To carry out research using the repertory grid test, the procedure must be taken a stage further.

5. Each of the people in the original list should be rated on each construct using a seven-point scale (see table 4.1).

6. The correlation coefficients (see above) between constructs are then calculated. If a pair of constructs correlate reasonably well, this means that different trait words

Table 4.1 Rating of constructs

Instructions: A list of constructs appears down the left-hand column. Rate each person on each construct using the numbers 1 to 7 where 1 means the person is entirely described by the adjective on the left and 7 means that the person is entirely described by the adjective on the right. For example, for the first construct, 'friendly–unfriendly', '1' means 'very friendly' and '7' means 'very unfriendly'. A score of 3 would mean that the person is neither very friendly nor very unfriendly.

Constructs	Father	Mother	May	Susan	Jane	John
Friendly–Unfriendly	3	1	5	2	3	2
Hard working–Lazy	1	3	5	6	3	4
Easily irritated–Placid	6	3	2	1	5	3
Sociable–Unsociable	4	2	1	4	6	2
Happy–Unhappy	3	4	5	3	2	1

are being used to describe the same underlying group of factors, or *factor constructs*. For example, 'easy to get on with' has a similar meaning to 'is friendly' and, if these two words are used in the same way, this indicates the existence of a construct 'easy to get on with/unfriendly'. The correlations between constructs will also identify factor constructs which do not correlate. These independent groups of constructs, the factor constructs, describe the underlying structure of the trait system used to judge other people.

Research with the repertory grid test shows that different people use different constructs. Moreover, some people use only a few independent constructs whereas others use many. Having only a few constructs is a sign of psychological immaturity, having many is a sign of psychological maturity.

Bias when judging others

There are several biases which occur when one tries to draw conclusions about others, whatever implicit personality theory is used. The result is that judging other people's personalities tends to be unreliable. A nurse alerted to these biases can improve her accuracy in assessing her patients' personalities.

Situation

The only way to judge personality is to look at behaviour. Behaviour results from an interaction between the person and the situation (see above).

Research shows that people tend to ignore the situation when judging another's personality (Jones and Nisbett, 1971). A good way to illustrate this is to compare the reasons given by a person for his own behaviour and the reasons given by someone else. If he is late for work, he is likely to explain his lateness in terms of some aspect of the situation: the alarm did not go off or the bus was cancelled. However, if someone else explains his lateness, they are much more likely to explain it in terms of personality characteristics: he is not careful enough or is not a punctual person.

To summarise the research findings, we tend to make external attributions (i.e. blame an aspect of the situation) for our own behaviour but internal attributions (i.e.

blame some aspect of personality) for the behaviour of others. Who is the more accurate, the person explaining their own behaviour or the person explaining someone else's behaviour? It is difficult to answer this question, but all that can be said is that people tend to ignore the situation when judging others.

A good nurse always looks for a situational explanation for a patient's behaviour. If patients are behaving oddly, it may not be their personality, but something in the situation, which is causing the problem. The word 'situation' should be interpreted in a very broad sense and should include anything which is not part of the person. For example, the situation may include the patient's medicines; some people behave oddly because of the drugs they are taking or because they are being withdrawn from drugs.

When people become patients, they find themselves in a different situation from that with which they are familiar. Some people react very badly to this and most people become more irritable when they are in pain or are anxious. It is unfortunate that nurses often see people at their worst, and allowances should be made for the effect of illness on a person's behaviour.

Some patients are labelled 'difficult'. Stockwell (1972) suggests that the difficult patient is one whose needs are not being met. Too often difficulties arise because nurses are unaware of the way in which a patient is reacting to a particular situation.

● Peter Farnsworth (aged 25) was admitted to hospital for treatment and placed in a side ward. He was told that the treatment was minor and that he would be out in a matter of days. However, complications arose and he had to remain in for more tests. The doctor assured him at every meeting that everything was all right. Peter realised that this was not so because his treatment was deviating from its original plan. He kept asking for more information but was still told by both doctors and nurses that everything was all right. Peter became more insistent on gaining information and the nurses began to avoid him because they did not know what to say. He became more angry and agitated with his treatment and berated anyone who came into his room. Soon the nurses saw as little as possible of Peter and new nurses on the ward were warned about him being a 'difficult patient'. There is a happy ending to the story: a student nurse who had been to a lecture on the 'difficult' patient decided to put into practice what she had learned. She went to see Peter, found out what was upsetting him and obtained some accurate information from the doctor. As a result, Peter stopped being 'difficult'.

Repeated observation

People's behaviour tends to vary over time and place. Some people are very irritable and unsociable when they first get up in the morning. And we all have 'off days' when we are not as friendly to other people around us as usual.

When making an assessment of another's personality, it is important not to make the assessment on the basis of just one observation, yet this is often precisely what people do when judging another. There are three biases which result from this: the first impressions effect, the recency effect and overgeneralisation across situations.

1. *First impressions effect*: People form impressions of others very quickly. Research reviewed by Schmitt (1976) shows that in interviews decisions are often made within the first four minutes. And, once a person has made an assessment, he is often reluctant to change his mind. Why is this? The reason for this is that forming

an assessment is equivalent to making a hypothesis, and we all like to see our hypotheses proved correct. Therefore, if we see someone behaving differently on a subsequent occasion we tend to reinterpret that behaviour to make it consistent with the first impression.

● Mrs Wilkins was admitted to hospital after several cancellations by the hospital of her earlier admission bookings. These cancellations had led to unnecessary inconvenience to Mrs Wilkins' friends who were going to help out while she was in hospital. Mrs Wilkins wanted to impose as little as possible on her friends and was annoyed by the cancellations. On admission, she made several disguised derogatory remarks to the nurses about the cancellations (e.g. 'It's just as well you're not running a business here'). The nurses were not paying proper attention to what Mrs Wilkins said and decided that she was a 'demanding patient'. Mrs Wilkins was subsequently given very little attention by the nurses on the ward. Whenever she tried to enter into a conversation, the nurses interpreted this as the prelude to 'yet another demand'.

2. *Recency effects*: There is a second time-based bias of person perception. In judging another overemphasis tends to be placed on what the person was doing when last seen, i.e. on what happened recently.

   The recency effect shows that the nurse will tend to remember the patient as she saw him most recently, and the first impressions effect show that she tends to remember the patient as she first saw him. There is a parallel between this and what was shown in chapter 3: that patients remember best what they are told at the beginning and the end of an interview. For both patients and nurses, beginnings and endings are remembered better than what happens in the middle.

3. *Overgeneralisation*: A third bias occurs because people overgeneralise the assessment of personality made in one situation to other situations. Some people behave quite differently in a ward situation than they do at home. For example, elderly people sometimes appear quite confused on admission to a ward, but are in fact perfectly rational in their home environment. At the beginning of the chapter, personality was defined as behaviour which is consistent across different situations. In assessing personality, the nurse must check that the behaviour which used to infer personality is actually consistent across different situations.

Good is not always beautiful

Patients are more likely to be convinced about an argument which is presented by an attractive communicator (see chapter 3). The reason behind this effect is the 'beautiful is good' bias. Nurses, like anyone else, are likely to be affected by the 'beautiful is good' bias in judging patients.

   Research reviewed by Darbyshire (1986) shows that there are several ways in which physical appearance affects attitudes towards and treatment of patients. For example, an attractive child who causes a disturbance is less likely to be blamed for the disturbance than an unattractive child. Parents are more likely to have positive expectations about an attractive baby than an unattractive baby, an expectation which may then become a self-fulfilling prophecy. Other research (described in Darbyshire, 1986) shows that unattractive patients are more likely to be rated as suffering from epilepsy or mental handicap than attractive ones, and are assumed to have a worse prognosis.

It is important that nurses avoid judging personality on the basis of physical appearance. Unattractive patients can be just as 'good' as attractive patients, and attractive patients are not always 'good'.

Stereotyping

A stereotype is a judgment which is made on the basis of very little evidence; the beautiful is good bias is a kind of stereotype. Stereotyping is a normal phenomenon —we all do it—but it can distort the truth. The way this distortion works is as follows. If objects or people are divided into groups and given labels, the very fact of giving a label distorts perception so that there is a tendency to overemphasise:

- The similarities within groups
- The differences between groups

For example, there is a label to describe a certain type of young person as a 'punk'. Seeing someone with spiky black hair and a safety-pin through his nose may lead to that person being labelled 'punk'. The effect of that label is to bias perception so that he is perceived as being more similar to other 'punks' (e.g. being aggressive) and less similar to other people.

Stereotyping occurs with many different sorts of group and label. For example, labels are based on skin colour (black versus white), on religion (Protestant versus Catholic), on nationality (America versus Russia), on political persuasion (democrats versus communists), on social class (middle versus working class), on gender (male versus female), and on sexual preference (homosexual versus heterosexual). Of course, not everyone uses all these ways of grouping people, but most of us use some way of labelling people; some of the constructs we use to assess people (see above) may actually be stereotypes.

The consequences of stereotyping is that it is possible to misperceive a person's personality by assuming that he is more similar to a certain group of people than he actually is. For example, nurses are assumed to know about nursing so, when a nurse becomes a patient, she does not always receive the same level of support as other patients. The nurse-patient often does not have things explained to her, even though she may work in a different branch of nursing and not have the knowledge she is assumed by the other nurses to have.

Although nurses share all the stereotypes of other people, they have an additional way of labelling. They, and other health professionals, also categorise patients in terms of illness. There are several reasons why illness-types are used as labels: first, medical practice classifies people in terms of illness; second, people with the same illness tend to be located on the same wards (e.g. in a renal or cardiac unit).

Wattley and Muller (1984) give a good example of how illness type can affect perception of patients. Two groups of nurses were asked to make an assessment on a written description of a patient. The description of the patient was the same for each group except for one thing. In one group, the patient was identified as being treated for cirrhosis of the liver, in the other by a simple hernia repair. Cirrhosis is known to be associated with heavy drinking and it is easy to blame the patient for inducing his condition. The nurses were asked to rate the likely patient charateristics on a series of personality traits. The results showed that the nurses expected the patient suffering from cirrhosis to be:

● 'less cheerful, more unhelpful, more ungrateful, slightly more uncooperative, more difficult to talk to, more willing to accept treatment and less likely to exaggerate the extent of the illness than the same patient would be if suffering from a hernia.' (pp.61–62)

The tendency to judge (in a moral sense) patients by their illnesses and treat them in accordance with that judgment is by no means uncommon. Patients with illnesses which are perceived to be 'self-inflicted' are treated more negatively by some, but not all, nurses (Kelly and May, 1982). For example, patients with sexually transmitted disease or requesting an abortion are more likely to be treated in an unfriendly fashion. The tendency to judge negatively and so be unfriendly to patients also occurs where the patient has socially unacceptable patterns of behaviour.

● Daphne was a male transvestite, expecting to have sex change operation in due course, who was admitted to hospital with rotated testicles and, after some discussion by the hospital management, was admitted to a female ward. In bed Daphne wore a pink nightie but was distinguished by a deep voice and hairy chest. Many of the trained staff were unable to cope with this, avoiding both the patient and any eye contact. Daphne felt very isolated but was accustomed to this feeling. One student nurse was able to maintain her standard of care for the patient because she consciously applied her knowledge of communication skills (see chapter 2), despite personally having a negative attitude towards Daphne. And, because of the effective communication, her negative attitude towards the patient began to disappear. The student nurse was acting in a highly professional way by not allowing her personal feelings to affect the quality of care she was giving.

It is very difficult to overcome one's biases about particular types of people and particular types of illness, but two points may help. First, we are all likely to be guilty of some self-inflicted illness at some time in our life, whether it is through drinking or smoking or not eating the right sort of food. One would explain one's own lack of health care by referring to the situation, for example, lack of information at the necessary time. But the situation tends to be ignored when judging someone else: he is blamed for having a weak personality. If blame has to be apportioned, it should be to the situation and not the patient. Let us return to the example of the male transvestite. It may be that this person's sexual preference was the consequence of a particular genetic make-up. Is it really fair to blame him for his chromosome structure?

Ultimately, of course, there is a moral issue about the nature of nursing. Nurses should care equally well for all people, irrespective of class, creed, nationality, skin colour, or type of illness.

Accuracy of judging others

As shown above, there are several biases which are likely to make the judgment of personality inaccurate. The question of accuracy of judgment has been the subject of several different types of research study, though it is recognised that there are methodological problems with this research, such as, the meaning of 'accuracy' when judging personality (Cook, 1984). One way of addressing the issue of accuracy is to compare the conclusions drawn by different interviewers about the same interviewee.

Early research on the reliability of interviews (reviewed by Arvey and Campion, 1984) showed that interviewers often fail to agree about an applicant's characteristics. Better agreement is reached when interviewers work in interview panels rather than there being separate interviews, and when structured interviews are used. Of course, interview panels and structured interviews may lead to the interviewee behaving very differently than he would in a one-to-one and unstructured interview.

Research also shows, not surprisingly, that the interviewer's characteristics have an effect on the outcome of an interview, with interviewer–interviewee similarity leading to more positive evaluation.

The practical implications of this research are as follows.

- When several people make independent assessments of another person's personality they often disagree in their conclusions

- People behave differently when talking to one person than when talking to another.

The lesson to remember is: don't make hasty judgments about another person's personality, you may be wrong!

Research on the 'unpopular patient'

It is inevitable that some patients are more popular with nurses than others. Stockwell's pioneering study in 1972 was instigated in part because of the possibility that unpopular patients might be treated less well and therefore recover more slowly than popular patients. Since then, there has been an abundance of research examining the popular/unpopular patient issue. A useful review of this research was presented by Kelly and May (1982), and the following is a summary of some of the conclusions in that review.

There are a number of personality characteristics which make a patient unpopular, although whether these personality characteristics are accurately perceived is another matter. In various studies, unpopular patients have been found to be rated as:

- Aggressive, violent, and angry
- Wanting immediate satisfaction, constantly complaining, being demanding and attention-seeking
- Uncooperative, failing to accept the type of care given, failing to accept any care at all, failing to accept the dependency which sickness implies and refusing to accept that they are ill

By contrast, popular patients are rated as being understanding, amusing, optimistic, cheerful and grateful.

There are two points to notice about these characteristics. The first is that the unpopular patient is one who does not fit in with the roles and expectations of patients as imposed by nursing and medical staff. Second, the popular patient is one who makes the nurses feel good and is best able to satisfy the nurses' needs. Patients who cause the nurse to feel ineffective, angry or anxious are particularly resented by nursing staff.

This research shows that patient unpopularity is not just a characteristic of the patient: it is the result of the interaction between the nurse and the patient. It is the failure to comply with what the nurse wants which makes a patient unpopular. Kelly and May conclude: 'The good patient is one who confirms the role of the nurse; the bad patient denies that legitimation'.

Chapter 1 introduced the idea that hospitals are 'unpleasant places to be', in part because they require patients to forfeit control, which in turn leads to various psychological deficits. However, not everyone is happy to relinquish control and suffer psychological deficits; some people exhibit reactance under conditions of uncontrollability. Reactance means that the person has not given up but is trying to regain control of his circumstances.

Taylor (1986) characterises the 'good' patient as someone who exhibits the symptoms of helplessness. Feelings of anxiety and depression, powerlessness and fatalism are combined with behaviours of compliance, passivity, inability to remember information and failure to provide condition-relevant information. By contrast, Taylor characterises the 'bad patient' as someone who exhibits the symptoms of reactance. Feelings of anger, and suspicion regarding his condition, treatment and staff behaviour are coupled with complaints to staff, demands for attention, mutinous behaviour and possible self-sabotage. Such feelings are associated with physical changes such as the production of stress hormones which can delay recovery. (See also Raps et al, 1982).

Clearly, the labels of 'unpopular' and 'difficult' will continue to be used by nurses and continue to conflict with the egalitarian principles on which nursing is based. Five recommendations can be made to the nurse who finds herself dealing with an unpopular patient.

1. The nurse should look for situational factors which are making the patient engage in unpopular behaviour and; in particular, factors which may lead him to exhibit reactance.

2. She should examine her own reasons for reacting negatively to a patient.

3. Non-verbal and verbal communication skills can be used to give the patient positive rather than negative signals.

4. The nurse can discuss with other staff how they react to the patient and the reasons for their reactions.

5. Finally, the nurse should not feel guilty if she dislikes a patient, but be honest with herself. Personality clashes do occur, but the object of professional nursing is that no patient perceives that he is disliked by the nursing staff.

Summary

This section has focussed on how the layman makes personality judgments about others. Judging other people is far from reliable as impressions are biased by:

1. Failing to take the effects of the situation into account

2. Overgeneralising from one or a limited variety of meetings

3. Physical appearance

4. Stereotyping

A nurse has only her common sense and observation with which to judge a person's personality; this section shows that that common sense and observation may prove to be very unreliable.

SEXUAL BEHAVIOUR

It has been stated previously that, in some aspects, people are similar to some people but different from others, and this is particularly true of sexual behaviour. Indeed, sexual behaviour is much more variable than is often thought. To understand a patient's needs, a nurse must understand the patient's sexual needs. And to understand about sexual needs, it is also necessary to know something about sexual behaviour and its variations.

Variation in the pattern of sexual behaviour

Culture

Research by anthropologists (e.g. Ford and Beach, 1952) who have examined sexual behaviour in different countries shows that it is largely determined by the culture in which we live. People who live in different cultures engage in sexual behaviour in a variety of ways and find different physical characteristics to be sexually exciting. To take one example, kissing and fondling of breasts are normal patterns of sexual activity in Western society, but are by no means universal. Consider three South American tribes, the Sirioni, the Chorotoni and the Apinaye. Kissing is unknown among the Sirioni but mutual scratching and biting is frequent and found to be sexually arousing. The Chorotoni spit in their lovers' faces during intercourse and the Aponaye may bite their partners' eyebrows.

The physical characteristics (these usually refer only to the female) thought to be sexually attractive also vary between cultures and over time within a culture. For example, sometimes pendulous breasts are preferred, sometimes highly positioned breasts, sometimes thin ankles, sometimes fat calves. In our own society there are shifts in the preferred stature of women. Two hundred years ago the 'ideal' female figure was rather plump, as in the paintings of nudes by Reubens. Nowadays, a thinner figure is preferred, though the very thin 'Twiggy' look popular in the 1960s is probably now considered too thin and boyish.

Homosexuality is regarded in Western society as a deviant sexual behaviour which is 'unnatural'. But what precisely is meant by 'unnatural'? Ford and Beach examined 76 'preliterate' societies which might be considered more close to nature than Western society and found that in 35 per cent of this sample homosexuality was rare or absent whereas in the remaining 65 per cent it was normal and socially accepted.

The observed variety of sexual behaviour and preference has led anthropologists to put forward the social labelling view which states that 'no sexual act is intrinsically deviant'. This is not entirely true because one sexual act, that of incest between close relatives, is forbidden for the general population in all societies (although what exactly constitutes a 'close relative' does vary). However, it does make a general point in showing that the form that sexual behaviour takes is learned within a society, and there may well be sanctions to ensure that people maintain their own particular society's way of engaging in sexual behaviour.

The lessons for the nurse to learn from this are that she should not be surprised to find people engaging in what to her is 'unusual' sexual behaviour, and that she should try not to be judgmental about it.

Homosexuality

Homosexuality is one of the better known forms of sexual variation which often attracts disapproval in Western society. Although the data from questionnaire surveys can be criticised, the general consensus of opinion (Feldman and MacCulloch, 1980; Harmatz and Novak, 1983) is that 4 per cent of males and 1 per cent of females are exclusively homosexual, which means that these individuals obtain sexual arousal only from homosexual contact. However, up to 20 per cent of males and 4 per cent of females may have had some form of homosexual relationship during their lives. The incidence of these occasional homosexual relationships is much higher in adolescents and young adults than in older adults. Interestingly, in some preliterate societies, homosexuality among young males is seen as a normal part of growing up, whereas the mature adult is heterosexual. The reason for the gender and age differences in the pattern of homosexuality is not known.

Although heterosexuals may find it incomprehensible that others should actually want to engage in homosexual relations, it is important not to be judgmental. Homosexuals do not choose to be homosexuals but discover that they naturally are, just like heterosexuals discover that they only find members of the opposite sex to be sexually arousing.

Changes in sexual activity

The amount of sexual activity engaged in can vary both between people and during a person's lifetime, and changes differently for males and females. In this context, sexual activity is defined as behaviour leading to, or likely to lead to, an orgasm and is a general term which includes both sexual intercourse and masturbation.

Males

Although sexual activity in males sometimes occurs before adolescence, most sexual activity starts with the onset of adolescence and peaks some three or four years afterwards, at an age of 16 or 17. Questionnaire surveys (reviewed in Harmatz and Novak, 1983) show that young males have an orgasm (often through masturbation) on average five times per week. Sexual activity begins to decline in the early 20s, with a gradual decline over the rest of the person's life. Many males are impotent by the time they are 60, or engage in very infrequent sexual activity. These figures are only averages; there is considerable variation in sexual activity. Some young males masturbate twice a day, others only once a week, and some elderly men maintain a high level of sexual activity into their seventies.

Thus, the 'normal' pattern of behaviour for young men is to masturbate or engage in sexual intercourse about once a day. There is a strong need to engage in sexual activity, and men find it unpleasant if they are unable to obtain a sexual outlet; this then leads to feelings of restlessness and discomfort. From the point of view of nursing care, therefore, the nurse should expect young, or even elderly, men who are in hospital to masturbate. This is normally done discreetly, as the young man does not want to draw attention to himself.

As with homosexuality, masturbation is often disapproved of in Western culture. In the Victorian era infibulation devices (spiked rings) were strapped on to prevent boys from masturbating. Contrary to myth, masturbation does not cause blindness, insanity or poor health. Most married men masturbate as well as engage in sexual intercourse.

Females

The onset of sexual activity is much more gradual in females than males. Not only do females, on average, start sexual intercourse at an older age than males, but females also engage less in masturbation (Harmatz and Novak, 1983). Whereas most men will have masturbated by the age of 20, only about a third of females will have done so. Female sexual activity seems to be much more geared to relationships rather than to physical activity and, indeed, the occurrence of an orgasm in sexual intercourse in females is much more linked to the relationship than is the case with males. Not all women achieve an orgasm during sexual intercourse for this and other reasons which will be discussed later.

As with men, there is a considerable variation in female sexual activity. Some women start sexual intercourse at a very early age, and some will masturbate more frequently than some men. However, the average pattern is for women to engage in less sexual activity than men during the first 10 years after adolescence.

As noted above, men's sexual activity starts to decline in their early twenties, but the evidence seems to suggest that women's sexual needs do not decline. Although there is a decline in the frequency of sexual intercourse in women over the age of about 30, this is probably attributable to the waning powers of the male partner, who is usually of a similar age. For sexual activities which are not initiated by a male, there is no decline in sexual activity; for instance, masturbation is as frequent in late teens as in women of 50 or 60 years of age.

In general terms, sexual needs in males and females are poorly matched. Men peak too young and burn out too soon, leaving older women dissatisfied. This mismatch can lead to relationship problems.

Sexual advances to the nurse

It is important to realise that nurses can be sexually attractive to patients and, just as female nurses can be sexually attractive to male patients, male nurses (both young and older) can be sexually attractive, often to older women.

There is no one correct way of dealing with sexual advances. The correct way is the one which suits the nurse best, and it is important for her to make up her mind in advance how to deal with this type of situation to avoid panic or unprofessional behaviour.

Two ways of dealing with advances which might be considered are treating the advance as a joke, and pretending that the invitation has not been heard and responding with a distracting remark. This latter tactic can be helpful in avoiding hurt feelings. It is important to realise that sensitivity is needed in handling such situations.

Some, typically older, men make sexually explicit remarks or gestures specifically to shock or upset a nurse. Often this behaviour is due to lack of sexual self-esteem on the part of a man who finds that the only way to get a response to his sexuality is to shock. There are several ways a nurse might react to this situation, but the main objective is to try to appear unshocked. An authoritarian or lighthearted response, or some mixture of the two, may be used, for example, 'That's enough of that Mr Smith, you'll upset the other patients'. Again, the nurse should react to this kind of provocation in the way in which she feels most comfortable, but it is important to plan a strategy in advance.

Other areas that a nurse might like to consider are the temptation to respond positively to a patient's advance, and the morality of nurses helping people who are tion). In the last analysis, the sexual involvement of a nurse with a patient is unprofessional.

Human sexual response

Masters and Johnson (1966) divide human sexual response into four stages: excitement, plateau, orgasm and resolution.

Excitement

Sexual excitement leads in the male to erection of the penis and in the female to lubrication and extension of the barrel of the vagina. Both these response are automatic rather than under voluntary control, and can be brought about by a variety of stimulations, from reading erotic stories, seeing erotic pictures, or thinking erotic thoughts to physical stimulation of a variety of parts of the body, typically the insides of the thighs and the genital region.

Penile erection, however, occurs in circumstances other than sexual excitement. It occurs during dreaming sleep and sometimes during periods of extreme relaxation. If a nurse is bathing a male patient, it is by no means unusual for him to develop an erection, which may or may not be due to sexual excitement caused by the nurse and her actions. It is important that the nurse should prepare herself in advance for such situations. She should try to ignore the fact that the patient's penis is erect and carry on with her task. She should not make an issue of it nor embarrass the patient by referring to it. It is an everyday occurrence and not under voluntary control.

Plateau, orgasm and resolution

Continual sexual excitement leads to a high state of sexual arousal the *plateau* which, with continued stimulation, leads to an orgasm. Males have a shorter plateau phase than do females and therefore can have an orgasm before the female is ready. Orgasm in the adult male is followed by a rapid *resolution* phase when the penis returns to its normal, unerect state. Early orgasm on the part of the male may mean that the female does not achieve an orgasm. However, if the male does not have an early orgasm, the female is capable of having multiple orgasms. Interestingly, pre-adolescent boys also have the ability to achieve multiple orgasms, but this ability is lost at adolescence when the brain develops from a 'female' to a 'male' type under the action of the sex hormone, testosterone.

Plateau, orgasm and resolution for males and females are illustrated in figure 4.4.

One of the consequences of the differing sexual response patterns between males and females is that females can be left sexually unsatisfied by sexual intercourse with males. If this causes distress, the problem can be remedied to some extent by modifying sexual techniques. For example, the duration of pre-intercourse stimulation (foreplay) can be increased, the male can use distraction as a way of lengthening the onset of orgasm or one or other partner can engage in clitoral stimulation. An orgasm from stimulation of the clitoris often occurs more quickly than from vaginal stimulation.

Sexual problems

In the male, the major sexual problems are premature ejaculation and an inability to maintain an erect penis. A large component of these problems seems to be due to the sufferer associating sexual activity with anxiety, and therapy is designed to reduce this association. From the perspective of reversal theory, sexual problems arise when the person becomes telic rather than paratelic during sexual intercourse. In the paratelic state, the high arousal of sexual intercourse is experienced as excitement, but in the telic state the high arousal is experienced as anxiety.

In the female, the major sexual problem is vaginismus, where the walls of the vagina contract tightly and sexual intercourse is painful or impossible. Again, the problem has anxiety as a basis, and therapeutic techniques are designed to reduce the association between sex and anxiety.

Sexual problems can be very distressing for the people involved, who are often reluctant to discuss their problems with others, and the nurse should be aware of hidden messages indicating these anxieties. Sexual problems are quite amenable to therapy and sufferers should be advised to see a qualified sex therapist, a useful initial point of contact is a National Health Service clinical psychologist.

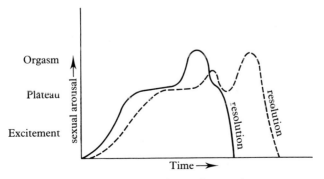

Fig. 4.4 Phases of sexual arousal

SUMMARY

The first part of this chapter provided an overview of theories of personality. These theories fell into four categories:

1. Need theories
2. Theories of intelligence
3. Trait theories
4. Reversal theory

These different theories were used to explore how different people need to be cared for in different ways.

The second part of this chapter showed how lay people make judgments about others' personalities. These judgments are affected by biases:

1. Failing to take the effects of the situation into account
2. Overgeneralising from one or a limited variety of meetings
3. Physical appearance
4. Stereotyping

Caution is needed when forming impressions of others, particularly when dealing with the 'difficult' patient. There is usually a reason why a patient is exhibiting difficult behaviour, and the good nurse should be able to find out what this is.

The third and final part of this chapter dealt with sexual behaviour and its variants. Nurses should prepare themselves to understand and manage human sexuality as a normal part of human behaviour.

References

Apter M J (1984) Reversal theory and personality: a review. *Journal of Research in Personality*, **18**: 265–288.

Arvey R D and Campion J E (1984) Person perception in the employment interview. In: *Issues in Person Perception*, ed. Cook M. London: Methuen.

Atkinson J W and Birch D (1978) *An Introduction to Motivation*. Princeton, New Jersey: Van Nostrand.

Bannister D and Fransella F (1971) *Inquiring Man: The Psychology of Personal Constructs*. Harmondsworth: Penguin.

Burger J M (1984) Desire for control, locus of control, and proneness to depression. *Journal of Personality*, **52**: 71–89.

Cook M (1984) The good judge of other's personality: methodological problems and their resolution. In: *Issues in Person Perception*, ed. Cook M. London: Methuen.

Darbyshire P (1986) When the face doesn't fit. *Nursing Times*, **82(39)**: 28–30.

Deci E L and Ryan R M (1985) *Intrinsic Motivation and Self-Determination in Human Behaviour*. New York: Plenum Press.

Eysenck H J (1952) *The Scientific Study of Personality*. London: Routledge & Kegan Paul.

Feldman P and MacCulloch M (1980) *Human Sexual Behaviour*. Chichester: John Wiley & Sons.

Ford C S and Beach F A (1952) *Patterns of Sexual Behaviour*. London: Methuen.

Harmatz M G and Novak M A (1983) *Human Sexuality*. New York: Harper & Row.

Henderson V (1966) *The Nature of Nursing*. London: MacMillan.

Hyland M E (1987) Control theory interpretation of psychological mechanisms of depression: comparison and integration of several theories. *Psychological Bulletin*, **102**: 109–121.

Jones E E and Nisbett R E (1971) The actor and observer: divergent perceptions of the causes of behaviour. In: *Attribution: Perceiving the Causes of Behaviour*, eds. Jones E E, Kanouse D E, Kelly H H, Nisbett R E, Valins S and Weiner B. Morristown, USA: General Learning Press.

Kelly M P and May D (1982) Good and bad patients: a review of the literature and a theoretical critique. *Journal of Advanced Nursing*, **7**: 147–156.

Kluckhohn C and Murray H A (eds.) (1953) *Personality in Nature, Society and Culture*. New York: Knopf.

Masters W H and Johnson V E (1966) *Human Sexual Response*. London: Churchill Livingstone.

Mathew A and Ridgeway V (1981) Personality and surgical recovery: a review. *British Journal of Clinical Psychology*, **20**: 243–260.

Murray H A (1938) *Explorations in Personality*. New York: Oxford University Press.

Raps C S, Peterson C, Jones M and Seligman M E P (1982) Patient behavior in hospitals: helplessness, reactance, or both. *Journal of Personality and Social Psychology*, **42**: 1036–1041.

Roper N, Logan W W and Tierney A J (1980). *The Elements of Nursing*. Edinburgh, London: Churchill Livingstone.

Schmitt N (1976) Social and situational determinants of interview decisions: implications for the employment interview. *Psychology*, **29**: 79–101.

Shackleton V and Fletcher C (1984) *Individual Differences: Theories and Applications*. London: Methuen.

Spearman C (1927) *The Abilities of Man*. London: Macmillan.

Stockwell F (1972) *The Unpopular Patient*. RCN Research Series. London: Royal College of Nursing.

Taylor S E (1986) *Health Psychology*. New York: Random House.

Wattley L A and Muller D (1984) *Investigating Psychology: A Practical Approach for Nursing*. London: Harper & Row.

Weiner B (1980) *Human Motivation*. New York: Holt, Rinehart & Winston.

White R W (1959) Motivation reconsidered: the concept of competence. *Psychological Review*, **66**: 319–327.

5

Caring for

Elderly People

The previous chapter showed that, while in some respects people are alike, in many other respects they are all different. This is just as true of elderly people as it is of any other age group so, in planning care for an elderly person, it is important to take account of the individual's needs, abilities and personality. To do this adequately, the nurse needs to understand the ways in which elderly people may differ from younger people. This chapter examines some of the psychological changes which are associated with ageing, and shows how elderly people may be helped to cope with these changes. It is important to remember that such changes do not affect all elderly people and that care must be individualised.

This chapter is divided into three main sections: the first part deals with some of the psychological changes associated with normal ageing, the second part examines the abnormal ageing processes which occur in people suffering from senile dementia and the third part provides an account of the psychological effects which may arise when elderly people experience a change in their circumstances, such as retirement or admission to an institution.

NORMAL AGEING

Two of the most important abilities in everyday life are communication and memory abilities. Both of these help us to feel in control of our lives and our environment. For example, communication helps us to make our desires known to other people, and so increases the likelihood that our wishes will be taken into account. Communication skills also enable us to understand the explanations which other people give us, and this makes events more predictable. Similarly, memory helps to increase predictability and control by enabling us to find our way around our environment, to know where we left our belongings and so on. In short, both communication and memory abilities help to enhance feelings of self-determination and so reduce the risk of learned helplessness (see chapter 1).

Communication

If an elderly person is having difficulty with communication, several problems may arise in addition to the feeling of reduced control. First, communication difficulties, the difficulties in exchanging messages, may lead to the elderly person becoming socially isolated. Social isolation can occur without physical isolation. Even when an elderly person is surrounded by other people, communication difficulties can create an invisible barrier which reduces or prevents social interaction. Second, communication difficulties may affect the way elderly people are perceived by other people. For example, they may be labelled as 'rude', 'unfriendly', 'stupid' or 'confused' when they are actually having difficulty in communicating. (This can be related to the discussion in chapter 4 of the 'difficult' or 'unpopular' patient.) The nurse can help alleviate some of these problems but, to do so, must understand the reasons why they have arisen: knowing what makes communication difficult is the first step towards making it easier.

There are three main causes of communication difficulty:

1. Problems with perception
2. Problems with attention
3. Problems with memory

For each type of problem there are several ways that communication can be improved by modification of verbal and non-verbal behaviour. These modifications supplement the basic communication skills which were introduced in chapters 2 and 3.

Problems with perception

Many communication problems in elderly people are due to perceptual problems. As people get older, their ability to perceive the world, especially through the senses of hearing and sight, tends to decline (see Kausler, 1982, for a detailed account).

One of the most common hearing disorders associated with age is *presbycusis*. A person suffering from presbycusis will have difficulty hearing quiet sounds, particularly if they are high pitched. This reduced auditory sensitivity will result in problems in perceiving speech. Some speech sounds, such as 's' and 'f', are especially likely to cause problems since they consist of high frequency sounds, and frequency is closely related to pitch.

Some elderly people find rapid speech particularly difficult to understand (Cohen, 1979). This is probably because of an age-related decrease in the speed with which the brain is able to process information. Botwinick (1978) has argued that successive speech sounds may become fused together in an elderly person's perception because the brain retains a record (a neural trace) of each sound for too long.

Failing vision may also reduce communication abilities. As shown in chapter 2, non-verbal communication can often be used to support or replace verbal communication. However, since many non-verbal cues are conveyed visually, an elderly person who has impaired vision may fail to pick up such cues. For example, facial expression can convey useful information about the meaning behind a verbal message: something said with a wink and a fleeting smile may mean exactly the opposite to the same thing said with a straight face. Therefore, if an elderly person misinterprets a statement, this may be because he has failed to pick up the subtle cues contained in the speaker's facial expression. People with hearing impairments are sometimes able to use lip-reading to compensate for their hearing loss but impaired vision reduces the feasibility of this strategy.

There are a number of ways to improve communication with elderly people who have perceptual problems.

1. Slow, clear and reasonably loud speech will help elderly people with hearing impairments. Shouting should be avoided as it is likely to distort the speech and may be painful to the elderly person's ears. Shouting can also give the impression that the speaker is angry even when he is not. It is important to adjust speech to suit the abilities of the individual listener: some elderly people may be offended if spoken to too slowly.

2. The pitch of the voice can be lowered slightly but should not be adjusted so much that it sounds unnatural.

3. Some speech sounds are more easily perceived than others. Therefore, if someone is having difficulty hearing a particular word, it is worth trying a different word with a similar meaning.

4. A posture should be adopted which enables the elderly person to see the speaker's face, and particularly lips, as clearly as possible. The person talking should also try to position himself in such a way that there is light shining on his face. This will help the elderly person to make use of lip-reading cues and cues from the facial expression.

5. A variety of senses can be used to present information. If an elderly person has problems with one sense (such as hearing), the nurse should make as much use as possible of other senses (such as sight and touch). For example, if a patient is having difficulty hearing the times at which she should take her medicines, writing the instructions down or drawing pictures of clocks showing the appropriate times may help. This is particularly important in a situation where an elderly patient is being prepared for discharge from hospital, or is in the community.

Problems with attention

There are two aspects of attention which are particularly relevant to communication: *selective attention* and *divided attention*. Selective attention is the ability to ignore irrelevant information and focus on the relevant information. For example, in order to understand a conversation, a person has to be able to focus his attention on what the speaker is saying without being distracted by background noise. Divided attention is the ability to attend to two different sources of information simultaneously or to do two different things at once. This ability is also important for communication. It enables listeners to understand a conversation even when two people are speaking at the same time, for example, when one speaker interrupts another. Also, divided attention allows a person to think about what he is going to say next and, at the same time, to listen to what another speaker is saying.

Research has shown that some elderly people's comprehension of speech is particularly badly affected by noisy conditions or by situations where several speakers are interrupting one another and speaking at the same time (Bergman, 1971; Corso, 1977). The communication problems experienced more severely by elderly than younger people in these conditions are likely to be due to difficulties with selective and divided attention. In other words, the elderly person has difficulty in filtering out background noise and in listening to two speakers at once. Kausler (1982) reports research evidence which indicates that as people get older their selective and divided attention abilities tend to decline. This evidence comes not only from tasks involving speech comprehension, but also from tasks involving perception of other types of sound and from visual perception tasks.

The nurse can help to reduce an elderly person's attention difficulties by several means.

1. Comments or questions should be addressed to an individual rather than to an entire group of people. This will help the elderly person to focus his attention on the speaker and on what is being said. This may sound time-consuming, but will probably save time in the long run, since it will increase the likelihood of the elderly person understanding what has been said, so will reduce the need for repeated explanation.

2. Eye-contact and touch may help to attract and maintain attention. Placing a hand on top of the listener's hand can be a useful way of aiding attention, especially if the elderly person has impaired vision. However, it is important to be sensitive to whether or not he finds the use of touch embarrassing (see chapter 2).

3. Background noise should be reduced as much as possible. The volume of the radio or television should be lowered, but the nurse should first check that the elderly person is not engrossed in a favourite programme.

4. Where several people are involved in a conversation, the extent to which they butt in and talk at the same time should be reduced. This will avoid the need for the elderly person to divide his attention between two speakers, so should make it easier for him to understand the conversation.

Problems with memory

Communication difficulties in the elderly may also be linked to memory problems. Memory abilities are discussed in some detail in the next section, and this section is restricted to those aspects of memory which are particularly relevant to communication.

In order to participate fully in a conversation involving several people, we need to remember not only what has been said earlier in the conversation but also who said what. Rabbitt (1981) carried out an interesting study which involved asking elderly people to remember either just the content of a conversation or both the content and which speaker had said what. The results indicated that the elderly people were good at remembering the content. However, when they were asked to remember both the content and who had said what, they found it difficult to recall either type of information. This suggests that trying to keep track of who has said what may interfere with remembering the content of a conversation. Rabbitt also found that when the subjects were asked to contribute their own comments to the conversation, their ability to remember other people's comments was reduced. These findings suggest that normal conversations may sometimes place severe demands on elderly people's memory abilities, although to some extent the difficulties experienced by Rabbitt's subjects may be related to the problems of attention discussed above. Again, there are ways of compensating for the effects of memory problems on communication.

1. If the nurse thinks an elderly person may have forgotten something which was said earlier in a conversation, the point can be reiterated. It is a good idea to express the statement in a different way the second time. This is known as *disguised repetition*. Disguised repetition should help reduce the risk of the elderly person perceiving the nurse's behaviour as patronising.

2. As with people who have attentional problems, the conversation should be structured to reduce butting in and overlapping contributions. This will make it easier for the elderly person to keep track of who has said what.

3. The carer needs to be sympathetic to the strategies which an elderly person may have developed to cope with difficulties in keeping track of complex conversations. These strategies may include engaging in monologue, making irrelevant remarks, failing to acknowledge other people's comments, or withdrawing from conversations altogether. A person who uses such strategies may be labelled as 'rude' or 'self-centred', but it is important to be aware that these strategies may indicate an underlying memory or communication problem. It may also be helpful to alert the elderly person's relatives to this possibility and to encourage them (tactfully) to react sympathetically to such behaviour.

Individualised care

This section has focused on some of the possible reasons for communication problems in elderly people, since an understanding of these contributes to an understanding of how to compensate for communication problems. However, it is important to remember that not all elderly people have communication problems. Also, the nature and extent of communication problems varies considerably from one old person to another. Several sorts of modification to verbal and non-verbal behaviour can help to compensate for communication difficulties, but these modifications should not be adopted automatically when talking to an elderly person. Instead, each individual's communication abilities should be continually monitored, and those particular modifications which seem to be appropriate to the individual selected. It is important to remember that people will usually communicate best about the topics which interest them most. Therefore, it is a good idea to try to find out about an elderly person's interests and bring these into the conversation. Asking to see photographs of family members or pets can be a useful starting point for a conversation.

Memory

Memory ability is an important component of people's ability to look after themselves. For example, self-care is unlikely to be successful if the patient does not remember instructions he was given or does not remember to carry them out (see chapter 3).

Memory ability is also important from the point of view of a person's feelings of competence and self-esteem. Persistent forgetfulness can lead to feelings of incompetence and low self-esteem: 'I'm useless. I'm always forgetting things'. Consequently, if people can be helped to remember, this may make them feel happier with themselves, as well as having practical benefits such as increasing the effectiveness of self-care.

Do elderly people have poorer memories than younger people? It is not possible to give a straightforward answer to this question. There is some evidence that, on average, older people's memory ability is less good than younger people's. However, there are at least three respects in which this statement needs to be qualified. First, there are considerable differences in memory ability within all age groups, including the elderly. Second, the memory abilities of different age groups overlap, so some elderly people have better memories than some young people. Third, elderly people's memory ability is more influenced by situational factors (such as the way information is presented and the way memory is tested) than is that of younger people. This means that the difference in memory ability between old and young people will be greater in some situations than in others. These situational variations (which form the focus of this section) provide useful clues as to how the elderly can be helped to succeed in remembering things. Most of the factors to be discussed affect memory ability at all ages, but their effect is particularly marked for elderly people.

Speed of presentation

One factor which influences memory ability is the speed at which the information to be remembered is presented. An elderly person is much more likely to remember information which is presented slowly than information which is presented at a rapid rate (Perlmutter and List, 1982). So, if the nurse is giving an elderly person self-care instructions which include several pieces of information, she should pay attention to the way she paces her explanation. It is not just the speed of speech which is important here, it is also important to consider the time interval between one piece of information and the next. There should be time for the listener to take in each point before going on to the next. If a complex procedure (such as care of a colostomy) is being taught, information should be spread over a number of sessions.

The above points would, of course, apply in situations where the communication is with a patient's elderly relatives.

Response time

Similarly, elderly people do better on memory tasks when they are given plenty of time to respond than when they feel that they are under pressure (Perlmutter and List, 1982). Therefore, if the nurse is asking a question which requires a person to remember something (e.g. 'What is your daughter's phone number?'), it is important to create a relaxed, unhurried atmosphere. It is possible to give the impression, through verbal and non-verbal behaviour, of being in a hurry when actually being perfectly prepared to wait for an answer. Being willing to spend time is not sufficient: this willingness must be communicated. Conversely, it is possible to convey the impression of having all the time in the world without actually spending a great deal of extra time. An unhurried atmosphere will increase the likelihood of the elderly person giving the correct information, so will probably save time in the long run. One way of creating an unhurried atmosphere is for the nurse to chat with the patient about something which is not directly relevant to the task in hand.

● *A hurried conversation*
  Nurse: Now, I want to find out certain things from you, Mrs Andrews, so we can plan your care. First, what is your daughter's phone number?

● *An unhurried conversation*
Nurse: Miserable day isn't it, Mrs Andrews? I don't like it when it rains, do you? (*Pauses for Mrs Andrews to reply*) By the way, could you tell me what your daughter's phone number is?

Recall versus recognition

Psychologists use different types of task to test people's memory ability. One particularly important distinction is between recall and recognition tasks. In a *recognition* task, the person is presented with some possible answers and has to decide whether each answer is correct or not. In a *recall* task, the person has to produce the correct answer from memory, without having a set of alternative answers to choose from.

The distinction between recall and recognition can be illustrated by the example of playing a party game similar to 'Kim's game'. First, a tray of assorted, small objects is shown and the players are asked to remember them. Then the tray of objects is removed and the contestants are given a test to see how well they can remember the objects. A recall test would require the listing of all the objects one could remember. In a recognition test, the original objects would be shown mixed in with some new objects and the task would be to pick out the objects which were seen earlier. In other words, the recall task requires the answer to the question: 'What was on the tray?', whereas the recognition task requires the answer to a series of questions of the form: 'Was this object on the tray?'. The recognition questions can be answered by 'Yes' or 'No', but the recall question cannot. Thus, the distinction between recall and recognition is closely related to the distinction between open and closed questions (see chapter 2).

People of all ages usually perform better in recognition tasks than in recall tasks, but this difference is even greater for elderly people than for younger people (Craik, 1977). Therefore, phrasing questions in such a way that tests for recognition rather than recall can help the elderly succeed in memory tasks. For example, if an elderly person seems to be having memory difficulties, the nurse might try asking, 'Did you leave your purse in your bedroom?', rather than, 'Where did you leave your purse?'.

Retrieval cues

People of all ages are likely to remember things better if they are provided with retrieval cues, such as, 'It begins with "m"' or, 'It's a kind of vegetable'. These retrieval cues seem to act like address labels; they direct the search of our memories. Again, there is evidence that retrieval cues are even more helpful to elderly people than to the young (Craik, 1977). If, for example, an elderly person is having difficulty remembering the nurse's name, she could try giving him a cue, such as the first letter, instead of telling him her name straight away. By using retrieval cues in this way, the chances of the elderly person successfully remembering facts will be strengthened, and his confidence in his own memory ability will be built up. Of course, if the elderly person does not give the correct answer in response to the retrieval cue, he should not be kept guessing for too long or his sense of failure will probably increase.

Cautiousness

Developing confidence in memory ability will often increase the likelihood of remembering information in future. In other words, there is a circular relationship between success and confidence: success increases confidence, which in turn increases success. One reason for this circular relationship is that the elderly tend to be more cautious than the young. Under many circumstances cautiousness is a good thing; for example, it can help prevent accidents. However, in a memory task, a cautious person may prefer to say, 'I don't know' rather than risk giving a wrong answer. If a person says, 'I don't know' in cases where he does know the answer but is not absolutely certain of this, he will appear to remember less than he actually does.

A study by Leech and Witte (1971) showed that when elderly people were rewarded for giving responses (irrespective of whether they were correct or not), their performance on a memory task improved. This suggests that cautiousness was masking their memory ability.

One way of reducing cautiousness is to try to ensure that the elderly person is not too anxious about a memory task. Too much anxiety interferes with people's ability to remember (see chapter 3), and this is particularly true of elderly people (Ross, 1968). Therefore, it is important to create a supportive context when asking an elderly person to remember something. For instance, the nurse should avoid showing any displeasure when an elderly person fails to remember something correctly, but should give praise when he succeeds. Discussions should take place in reasonable privacy and when the patient seems to be relaxed. The aim should be to encourage success, while reducing feelings of pressure and fear of failure.

Summary

Elderly people are most likely to remember information when:

- The information is presented reasonably slowly
- They are not rushed into giving an answer
- The questions test for recognition rather than recall
- Retrieval cues are provided
- Their anxiety is reduced, for example by support and encouragement

SENILE DEMENTIA

Dementia is a condition which involves deterioration of intellectual functioning. The deterioration is global rather than specific; that is, it affects many aspects of intellectual functioning. Also, the deterioration is progressive. As time goes on, the dementia becomes more severe, although the rate of deterioration varies from person to person. Dementia has a neurological basis, in that the deterioration of intellectual functioning is associated with pathological changes in the brain. The precise nature of these changes is as yet not fully understood and varies according to the type of dementia. Usually, the term 'pre-senile dementia' is used to refer to dementia occurring before the age of 65 years, and 'senile dementia' is used for dementia occurring at or after the age of 65.

How common is senile dementia? Kay and Bergmann (1980) estimate that 6.5 per cent of people over the age of 65 suffer from senile dementia, and that the percentage of sufferers increases to 17.7 for the over-80 age group. Most of the elderly people affected by dementia will be living in the community: Kay and Bergmann found that only about 25 per cent of moderately and severely demented people were living in institutions. These statistics show that dementia affects only a minority of the elderly population. Nevertheless, the absolute number of senile dementia sufferers—estimated as 700 000 in the UK (Holden and Woods, 1982)—is certainly not insignificant, and it can be assumed that this figure will rise considerably in the near future since the size of the elderly population as a whole is growing rapidly.

Although not all dementia sufferers will show exactly the same symptoms, it is possible to identify a range of symptoms which are characteristic of dementia. These characteristic symptoms fall into three categories (Gilleard, 1984):

1. Cognitive changes
2. Emotional changes
3. Behavioural changes

Cognitive changes

Cognitive changes are changes in a person's intellectual abilities, such as remembering, learning and thinking. Memory problems are among the most common and most obvious symptoms of dementia. In the early stages people typically have difficulty remembering information which they have recently encountered, but can usually remember information from the more distant past. Also, memory problems are especially likely to arise for abstract material and for material which does not have obvious personal relevance. However, in the later stages of dementia, even old and personally-relevant memories tend to be affected.

Dementia sufferers have problems not only with remembering factual information (such as people's names), but also with remembering the layout of the environment. Consequently, a person with dementia may have difficulty in finding his way around and may frequently get lost. This problem is particularly likely to arise in new, unfamiliar environments since memory loss is usually more severe for new memories than for older memories. For example, someone who is in the early stages of dementia may be able to find his way around his own home and neighbourhood, but may become disoriented when he has to cope with a new environment on admission to hospital.

There is another reason why dementia sufferers can have problems in finding their way around: dementia can interfere with people's ability to remember their own plans and intentions. For example, someone may leave his house with the intention of visiting the shops, but then forget where he was planning to go, and, therefore, wander aimlessly. This difficulty in remembering intentions does not only affect the intention to go somewhere; it can also affect the intention to do something.

If a dementia sufferer frequently forgets what he is trying to do, this is likely to result in him feeling that he is not in control of his own actions. In short, he may experience feelings of helplessness (see chapter 1). Furthermore, a person who cannot remember his own intentions is liable to suffer from self-neglect, since important activities such as eating, dressing and washing may be disrupted. Thus, the cognitive changes associated with dementia can bring about emotional changes (e.g. feelings of helplessness) and behavioural changes (e.g. self-neglect).

Emotional changes

Senile dementia does not produce a single type of emotional change: different people react in different ways. Some dementia sufferers experience feelings of depression, anxiety and agitation. It is probable that these feelings are at least partly due to the person's awareness of his declining competence and his declining control over his actions and environment. This interpretation receives some support from the results of a study which showed that depression is less common in severely demented people than in mildly demented people (Reifler, Larson and Hanley, 1982), as people who are only mildly demented are usually more aware of their condition than those with severe dementia.

Some dementia sufferers experience neither depression nor anxiety. Indeed, some may appear to be emotionally indifferent: they do not express feelings of happiness, sadness, fear or anger. Such people behave apathetically and find it difficult to take initiatives or to formulate their own plans. This difficulty (like the tendency to forget plans after they have been formulated) is likely to reduce the person's ability to carry out self-care activities.

Behavioural changes

Behavioural changes often accompany the onset of dementia. One of these changes, wandering and getting lost, has already been described as a consequence of memory problems. However, memory loss is not the only possible reason for wandering. In some cases, wandering may be due to a general feeling of restlessness and a desire for activity. There are also other behavioural changes which can affect dementia sufferers. Two of the most distressing of these are incontinence and aggressive behaviour.

Incontinence

Some dementia sufferers are affected by incontinence. Again, there is more than one possible reason for this. For example, it may be due to difficulty in remembering where the toilet is, or to difficulty in formulating and remembering the plan to visit the toilet. Alternatively, incontinence may be unrelated to the person's dementia; for instance, it may be due to a urinary tract infection or difficulty in walking so that the sufferer fails to reach the toilet in time.

Aggression

Sometimes, dementia is accompanied by an increase in aggressive or hostile behaviour. Sudden angry outbursts (which may seem to be unprovoked) can be very upsetting for carers, so it is important to understand some of the possible reasons for such behaviour. Aggression may sometimes be triggered by situations which make the dementia sufferer particularly aware of his declining competence. For example, an offer of help may be interpreted as a threat to the person's independence and may serve as a reminder of his declining ability. It is not uncommon for a dementia sufferer to accuse other people of stealing or hiding his possessions. Such accusations may help to protect the person with dementia from the painful knowledge that his memory is deteriorating and that his control of his own environment is diminishing.

● Mrs Walker suffers from senile dementia. She lives with her husband in their own home. Their daughter, Susan, and her husband, Andrew, live nearby and visit regularly. Mrs Walker is always mislaying her belongings, and becomes frustrated when she cannot remember where things are. On one occasion, she noticed that her engagement ring was not on her finger. Her husband asked where she had left it and she said she was sure she had left it next to the sink. But the ring was not there. Mrs Walker suddenly burst out: 'Andrew must have taken it. I always knew he couldn't be trusted. Lots of other things have been disappearing too—money, cutlery, all sorts of things'. Mr Walker was very upset, as both he and Mrs Walker had always got on very well with their son-in-law, and he could not understand why Mrs Walker had become so hostile towards Andrew. Fortunately, Mr Walker managed to dissuade his wife from confronting Andrew and Susan with the accusation. Mrs Walker's ring turned up the next day on the sitting room mantelpiece.

Caring for people with dementia

Self-care

People with dementia, like other patients, will benefit from opportunities to engage in self-care. Indeed, denying the patient the opportunity to engage in self-care should be avoided, as one way of implying that a person lacks competence is to do everything for him. Situations which highlight a dementia sufferer's competence can trigger aggressive behaviour, which suggests that encouraging dementia sufferers to engage in self-care might reduce aggressive behaviour. Furthermore, the risk of learned helplessness is likely to be reduced if self-care is encouraged.

However, the situation is complicated in that dementia reduces the extent to which a person is capable of self-care, so encouraging self-care can sometimes highlight the person's declining competence. The nurse is faced with a dilemma: is it better to do everything for the person (which implies that he is incompetent) or to allow the person to care for himself (which is likely to lead to him experiencing failure and thus to a feeling of incompetence)? The ideal solution to this dilemma is to ensure that each individual engages in as much self-care activity as is within his capabilities so that he experiences success but not failure. In practice, it can be difficult to achieve this solution, but it is an excellent goal to work towards.

Individualised patient care

Individualised patient care is essential in order to gear the amount of self-care activity to the person's level of competence. As part of individualised care, the nurse should assess each individual's abilities and use the results of the assessment to plan appropriate care. Sandman et al (1986) describe how this approach can be applied in the care of patients with dementia. On the basis of Orem's model (Orem, 1980), they argue that the goal of nursing should be to compensate for any lack of self-care ability. For example, one of the patients they studied had difficulty initiating actions (such as washing his hands) but he was able to complete an action if someone started it off for him. Thus, a nurse could compensate for this patient's lack of self-care ability by guiding his hands to begin with and then letting him finish off the action for himself.

Communication

Dementia (especially if it is severe) can interfere with the sufferer's sense of personal identity and ability to maintain social relationships. This, in turn, may make it difficult for carers to communicate with the patient and to treat him as an individual who has psychological needs. An interesting study by Armstrong-Esther and Browne (1986) found that nurses communicated less with confused than with lucid elderly patients. Armstrong-Esther and Browne suggest that this may be because communication with confused patients seems less rewarding.

Yet, ironically, the confused patients are the ones who are most in need of good communication as a means of contact with reality. For all of us, communication is crucial for keeping in touch with external reality. By communicating, we can find out about other people, about events which we have not experienced or have forgotten, and about what may be going to happen in the future. If we did not communicate, we would have to rely completely on our own experiences and memories, and this would result in our having a very narrow and distorted view of reality. This situation is likely to be exaggerated in the case of dementia sufferers, since their memory ability is declining. In other words, if they are deprived of opportunities for communication, it is highly probable that their confusion will increase. On the other hand, if communication between patients with dementia and their carers can be improved, some of their symptoms may be reduced.

Reality orientation

One approach which aims to improve communication with dementia patients is reality orientation (RO). As its name suggests, the central aim of reality orientation is to orient the elderly person to current reality, to increase his awareness of who he is, where he is (in place and time) and what is happening in his surroundings. There are two main ways in which RO tries to achieve this aim: by adopting a special approach to communication and by providing a structured environment. In practice, these two components of RO should be combined, but we shall consider them separately for the sake of clarity.

The RO approach to communication involves making a deliberate attempt to communicate with the dementia sufferer about current reality. Thus, basic information about names, dates, times and current events is presented as frequently as possible. However, it is not enough just to present such information; it is important also to try to ensure that the elderly person understands what is said and plays an active part in the conversation. The techniques introduced earlier in this chapter for improving communication and memory are useful for improving communication with dementia sufferers. It is also important to encourage the elderly person to repeat the information about current reality and to respond to what is being said.

Another principle of the RO approach to communication is that confused, rambling talk should be discouraged. Holden and Woods (1982) suggest three possible strategies for handling rambling talk:

1. Tactfully disagreeing and gently correcting what the patient says, for example: 'Well, actually I'm a nurse, but I do look quite like your daughter'.

2. Using distraction. This might involve changing the topic of conversation or drawing the patient's attention to something in the immediate environment.

3. Ignoring the content of the rambling talk but acknowledging the feelings expressed. For example, an elderly patient who does not want to get up at the time dictated by hospital routine might say, 'I've got to stay in bed until my mother comes and tells me it's time to get ready for school'. An appropriate response from a nurse would be, 'Are you feeling tired? Would you like to stay in bed for a little longer this morning?'.

The choice of strategy will depend on the situation and the individual. The important point is that all these strategies provide a way of avoiding agreeing with rambling, inaccurate talk.

The second component of reality orientation is the use of a structured environment to help the patient's memory and awareness of current reality. Signposts can be used to help him find his way around; for example, large arrows on the floor or walls could be used to guide people towards the toilets. Similarly, the doors to different rooms could be painted in different colours to help people to distinguish between them, or differently coloured signs could be used for the different rooms.

There are various ways of helping patients with dementia keep track of time. These include the use of clocks, calendars and diaries. A special notice-board can be used to display such information as the day, date, season and weather.

However, it is not sufficient merely to provide a structured environment. Steps should be taken to help the patient benefit from the environmental cues.

1. Memory aids (such as clocks and calendars) should be large and clear so that they can be seen easily even by people with impaired vision.

2. It is crucial that the information provided on boards, clocks and calendars is accurate and up-to-date; otherwise, it will increase rather than decrease the patients' confusion.

3. Patients' attention should be drawn to memory aids and environmental cues during conversation and they should be encouraged to use these cues. Begert and Jacobsson (1976) found that patients with senile dementia did not benefit from environmental cues unless they were actually taught to make use of them.

This brings us to the issue of the effectiveness of reality orientation: does it actually work? Although this may appear to be a simple question, it is in fact very complex. In the first place, the answer to this question will depend on how we define the criteria for success. How do we decide whether or not RO has worked? Since senile dementia involves progressive deterioration and since there is no known cure for senile dementia, it would be unrealistic to expect dramatic improvements in a patient's condition. Thus, a slowing down in the rate of deterioration may be evidence that RO is having a beneficial effect. In the second place, the answer to the question, 'Does RO actually work?' will depend on exactly how it is carried out. Reality orientation is not just a method of care but a philosophy of care, and the way it is carried out will vary according to the attitudes of the staff. Furthermore, RO includes a wide range of different techniques and activities so the particular elements which are used will vary from one ward or nursing home to another, and these variations need to be taken into account when assessing the effectiveness of RO.

Studies which have attempted to evaluate the effectiveness of RO have not produced a simple, consistent answer to the question of whether or not it works. This is not particularly surprising in view of the complexities already discussed. However, there is evidence which suggests that RO is most likely to be effective when it is adapted to suit the particular setting in which it is being used (Burton, 1982) and when it is adapted to the needs of individual patients (Adams, 1986). Thus, RO should not simply be treated as a 'package' which can be applied in the same way to all individuals in all settings. Instead, each patient's needs should be assessed and this assessment should form the basis for individually-planned care. Reality orientation provides a guiding framework and a useful pool of ideas and techniques which can be drawn on when planning the care of an individual patient.

CHANGES IN CIRCUMSTANCE

Throughout our lives we all experience various changes in our circumstances such as leaving school, getting married or moving home. These changes will often affect our behaviour and our feelings, although it is sometimes difficult to distinguish between the effects of changes in circumstance and the effects of growing older. For example, consider the case of a 25-year-old, married man who behaves more responsibly than he did when he was 18 and unmarried. Is the increase in responsibility due to the man being married or is it due to him being older? The most likely answer is that it is due to a combination of these two factors. This same principle applies to elderly people. In other words, the effects of growing old and the effects of changes in circumstance are intertwined. This section focuses on some of the changes in circumstance which elderly people may experience.

Living in an institution

Some elderly people will experience the change of moving from their own or a relative's home into an institution, such as a hospital or nursing home. Of course, it is not only elderly people who live in institutions and many of the points made in this section could be applied to people in any age group. However, there are two main reasons for discussing institutional care in this chapter. First, a large proportion of the people who are receiving institutional care are elderly. Second, some of the effects of living in an institution may be misinterpreted as effects of ageing.

Living in an institution can have a number of advantages for an elderly person. Financial or health problems sometimes make it difficult for elderly people to look after themselves adequately in their own homes, and these people are likely to benefit from the support which institutional care can provide. For example in a hospital or residential home elderly people are provided with a warm environment and regular hot meals without having to worry about the electricity or gas bill. Also, institutional care can provide elderly people with opportunities for social interaction, opportunities to talk to others and make new friends. This can be a particular advantage for a previously housebound person who did not have many visits from friends or relatives. Another advantage of institutional care is that it can relieve the feelings of guilt which many old people have about being a burden to their relatives: an elderly person may prefer to live in an institution rather than to live with a relative.

Despite the advantages of institutional care, there are several possible disadvantages. Institutions can have adverse effects on psychological well-being. These adverse effects are not inevitable and can be avoided or reduced by adapting the care to the patient's needs. There are four main types of adverse effect:

1. Confusion and disorientation
2. Learned helplessness
3. Social withdrawal
4. Depersonalisation

Confusion and disorientation

Confusion has already been discussed in relation to senile dementia. However, it is important to realise that confused behaviour does not necessarily indicate that an elderly person is suffering from dementia. Most people can remember an occasion when they were in an unfamiliar environment, for example, a first day at school or college, and the associated feeling of disorientation in such a situation. Even if one does not actually lose one's way in a new place, there is often a feeling of great anxiety about the possibility of doing so. Imagine how much worse this disorientation and confusion would be when feeling ill or with impaired vision or hearing. Thus, it is not surprising that elderly people sometimes experience confusion and disorientation on admission to hospital. This can be intensified if a patient's bed is moved to a new position in the ward, and this should be avoided where possible.

Although confusion is not always due to senile dementia, some of the techniques used to care for patients with dementia are also useful for reducing confused behaviour in those not suffering from dementia. In particular, clear communication and environmental cues will help to reduce confusion. Elderly people should be given clear explanation about who the carer is, why they are in the institution, the activities and facilities available, and so on. In doing this, it is important to follow the guidelines for improving communication outlined earlier in this chapter. Environmental cues such as signposts are also useful in reducing confusion. It is important that these are large and clear so that they can be read easily by people with deteriorating sight.

One reason why institutional environments may be confusing is that they often lack variety: every ward or room looks the same; all the corridors look the same; all the beds in a ward look the same. This makes it difficult for patients or residents to learn their way around and to work out where they are should they get lost. Although a nurse will have only limited control over the design of the institutional environment, she should try to introduce as much variety as possible. For example, patients could be encouraged to display their own possessions. Wards can be made much more cheerful and interesting by colourful pictures and soft furnishings, and many patients would enjoy making these articles themselves. Some areas operate a 'picture loan' scheme which enables hospitals and homes to borrow pictures to brighten up the walls.

Learned helplessness

If people feel that they are not in control of what happens to them, then they can experience learned helplessness (see chapter 1). In some institutions, elderly people are given very little control over their experiences and environment. The staff do everything for them: they wash them, dress them, feed them, make their beds, take them to the television room, put them to bed and so on. Everything follows a rigid timetable. All the patients are having the same things done to them at the same time every day. There is very little need, or opportunity, for the residents to make any decisions or choices, and they are encouraged to be passive and dependent on the nurses. The ward routine is seen as being more important than the patients as individuals. In such circumstances, there is a considerable risk that patients will learn to be helpless.

Learned helplessness affects motivation. People become apathetic and stop trying to do things for themselves because they have learned that they are not in control of events. The fact that patients then sit around doing nothing is likely to reinforce the nurses' belief that they are not capable of doing anything for themselves. In addition, learned helplessness can reduce people's cognitive ability and self-esteem, and can make them feel sad or depressed.

In order to reduce the risk of learned helplessness, it is important to give elderly people as much choice and control as possible. The effectiveness of such an approach is strikingly demonstrated by a study which Langer and Rodin (1976) carried out in a nursing home for elderly people. Langer and Rodin arranged for two similar groups of residents to be treated differently. The residents in one group (the 'responsibility-induced' group) heard a talk in which a senior member of staff stressed that the residents were responsible for the way they led their own lives. These residents were encouraged to make various choices and decisions about how to spend their time. Also, they were given the opportunity to choose a pot-plant, and were told that it was their responsibility to look after the plant in whatever way they thought best. The residents in the other group (the 'comparison' group) also heard a talk from the same member of staff, but this time the speaker stressed that it was the staff's responsibility to run the residents' lives. Both groups were told that the staff wanted them to be happy but the crucial difference between the two talks concerned whose responsibility it was to make the residents happy. The residents in the comparison group also received pot-plants. However, they were not given the opportunity to choose which particular plant they wanted, and they were told that the nurses would look after the plant for them. Langer and Rodin found that, three weeks after hearing the talk, the residents in the responsibility-induced group were happier, more alert and more active than the residents in the comparison group. In other words, the responsibility-induced residents showed less evidence of the affective, cognitive and motivational deficits associated with learned helplessness. The change which Langer and Rodin introduced into the elderly people's environment, although slightly more than described above, was actually quite minor. Nevertheless, this change had a considerable effect on their psychological well-being. If elderly patients are allowed as much choice, control and independence as possible, the results are likely to be even more dramatic.

Social withdrawal

Although living in an institution can sometimes provide increased opportunity for social interaction, this potential benefit does not always occur. In some residential homes and wards for the elderly, there is very little social interaction either among the residents themselves, or between the elderly people and staff. For instance, the residents may spend most of their time sitting in their favourite chairs (or the chairs in which they have been placed that day), watching television or gazing into space, and there may be very few conversations or social activities. Similarly, interactions between staff and residents may be restricted to brief communications about routine aspects of care (Lipman et al, 1979).

There are several possible reasons for elderly people becoming socially withdrawn. Cumming and Henry (1961) put forward the 'disengagement theory' which claims that social withdrawal (or *disengagement*) is an inevitable consequence of ageing. According to this theory, the elderly person chooses to step back from social activities, and society as a whole moves away from the elderly person. Furthermore, supporters of this theory argue that disengagement is necessary for the elderly person's psychological well-being. Disengagement is seen as successful adjustment to old age.

However, disengagement theory has been challenged, and some people have put forward precisely the opposite theory: that the people who adjust successfully to old age are those who remain active and socially involved (Atchley, 1976; Rhee, 1974). This is known as the 'activity theory'.

Evidence from research (Neugarten, 1977) indicates that, whereas the disengagement theory is true for some elderly people, the activity theory applies to others. Different people have different strategies for adjusting to old age, which are related to differences in personality. On the whole, an individual's personality is consistent throughout the life-span. Thus, extroverts (see chapter 4) will tend to continue to enjoy socialising as they grow older, whereas introverts may prefer a certain amount of social withdrawal. The implication of these differences is that elderly people living in institutions should be allowed to choose the extent to which they participate in social activities. Opportunities for social interaction and activity should be provided, but it should not be assumed that everyone will always want to take part. Likewise, not all elderly people are alike, and it should not be assumed that an elderly person will make the same choices every day. Even if he does not want to take part in an activity today, he should still be invited to do so tomorrow.

How can opportunities for social interaction be provided? One important consideration is the layout of the environment. For example, Peterson et al (1977) found that there was more social interaction among elderly patients when their chairs were arranged in small groups around tables, than when all the chairs were arranged side-by-side around the walls of a room. This result is not surprising given the importance of eye contact and facial expression in communication (see chapter 2). It is much easier to make use of these non-verbal signals when sitting at an angle to someone rather than side by side.

Another way of encouraging social interaction is to introduce activities which have a clear purpose and are meaningful to the residents. Such activities can provide a focus and a reason for social interaction. The sheltered workshop approach aims to encourage elderly people to participate in useful activities. For example, MacDonald and Settin (1978) describe a workshop which involved elderly residents making gifts for children in a nearby residential school. In addition to making the gifts, the elderly people met the children to hand over the completed presents. MacDonald and Settin found that the residents who took part in the workshop became more socially involved than another group of residents who did not have the opportunity to participate, but who had been comparable to the workshop group at the beginning of the study.

Giving elderly people independence and control can also encourage sociability. For example, Gustafsson (1976) found that social interaction improved when elderly patients were allowed to help themselves to coffee instead of being served by the nurses.

Depersonalisation

The term 'depersonalisation' refers to feelings of loss of dignity and self-esteem. Such feelings are likely to occur in institutions where people are not treated as individuals with psychological needs. In other words, the risk of depersonalisation is greatest when all patients or residents are treated in the same way and when staff concentrate on providing physical care to the exclusion of psychological care.

The risk of depersonalisation can be reduced by encouraging independence and social interaction in the ways described above. There are also a number of other steps which can be taken to avoid depersonalisation, such as:

1. Respecting the elderly person's privacy, for example, by providing screens when he is dressing or undressing

2. Encouraging the display of personal possessions and allowing the room or area of the ward to be arranged according to personal taste

3. Letting elderly people wear their own clothes rather than those provided by the institution

4. Not calling the elderly person by his first name unless he asks the nurse to do so; using an elderly person's first name without permission implies that he is being treated as a child

5. Not talking to others about the elderly person in his presence as if he was not there, since doing so suggests that the patient cannot understand; instead, the elderly person should be involved in the conversation

6. Chatting with the elderly person. This will help to build up a relationship by finding out about the elderly person's likes, dislikes and interests. Many elderly people enjoy giving their life histories and these can help the nurse to understand each person as an individual. Giving an account of his past history can also help an elderly person's self-esteem, as self-esteem in this age group derives largely from the past, rather than from the present or future. It is important to remember that chatting with a patient is not wasting time; it is a very important aspect of care.

Treating an elderly person in the ways just described will convey a very important message about the nurse's attitude towards him: that she respects him and is interested in him as an individual. This message is an excellent antidote to depersonalisation.

Retirement

Although not all retired people are elderly and not all elderly people are retired, many elderly people in the UK are retired. In order to provide good care for the elderly, it is important to understand the ways people react to the changes in circumstance associated with retirement.

As with most changes in circumstance, people react to retirement in different ways. For some, retirement represents a change for the better, while for others it represents a change for the worse. In other words, retirement can lead to either advantages or disadvantages and, indeed, many retired people experience a mixture of both advantages and disadvantages (Parker, 1982).

A large-scale survey carried out in Britain in 1977 revealed that, although people differ considerably in their experiences of retirement, it is possible to identify some recurrent themes (Parker, 1982). There are certain experiences which are commonly associated with retirement, but different people will have different combinations of these (and some retired people may not have any of the 'common' experiences). These experiences can be divided into two categories:

1. Gains or advantages
2. Losses or disadvantages

Gains

The main gain reported by retired people was a feeling of increased freedom. This took two main forms which Parker summarises as 'freedom to' and 'freedom from'. Retirement can increase a person's freedom to do as he wishes since it typically provides him with more leisure time than he had previously. Thus, for example, a retired person may benefit from opportunities to take up new hobbies, to spend more time on existing hobbies, to spend more time with his family or to spend more time relaxing. Retirement can also bring freedom from the unpleasant aspects of work. The extent to which a retired person experiences this feeling of freedom will obviously depend on his previous experience of, and attitude to, work. Some retired people experience feelings of freedom from the pressures of a stressful job, whereas others are pleased to be free from the rigid timetables imposed by their jobs, having to get up early and having to eat meals at set times, for example.

Losses

Financial loss: For most people, retirement brings a drop in income and so involves financial loss. Lack of money can limit the extent to which retirement provides the individual with freedom to do as he wishes. As one would expect, lack of adequate income tends to reduce satisfaction with retirement (Friedmann and Orbach, 1974). On the other hand, retired people who are financially comfortable do not always adjust well to their retirement (Beveridge, 1980).

Loss of social contact: Another loss commonly experienced by retired people is the loss of social contact. Many jobs provide the opportunity to interact with other people and to develop relationships with colleagues, customers or clients. Retirement typically involves severing (or at least weakening) many of the social relationships which have developed in the work context, and this can result in a sense of loss. Indeed, when the retired people in Parker's survey were asked what they missed most, the most common reply was, 'The people at work'. In addition to this particular factor, retired people sometimes feel deprived of opportunities for social contact and social interaction and, consequently, experience feelings of isolation and loneliness.

Role loss: Many people see their jobs as providing them with a specific role in society and therefore a usefulness which may disappear after retirement. Additionally some retired people miss the routine associated with work. They feel that they have too much time to fill and feel bored. Having more time available for leisure activities is not always regarded as a benefit.

Job loss: At a superficial level, the most obvious loss associated with retirement is the loss of the job itself. However, from a psychological point of view, this is often not perceived as being the most significant loss. In Parker's survey, only 11 per cent of retired people said that the work itself was what they missed most, whereas 36 per cent said, 'The people at work' and 31 per cent said, 'The money the job brought in'.

Helping people adjust to retirement

It is important to note that several of the losses experienced by retired people are not inevitable consequences of retirement. In particular, it is possible to avoid or reduce retired people's feelings of loneliness, boredom and uselessness. One way of doing this is to provide appropriate facilities for retired people and to ensure that they are informed of the opportunities which are available. For instance, sheltered workshops can be valuable in a community setting as well as in an institutional setting. A wide range of leisure and educational facilities should be provided for retired people so that each individual can choose activities which suit his interests.

In recent years, the importance of preparing people for their retirement has been increasingly recognised. A certain amount of retirement preparation is carried out by some employers, by local education authorities, by agencies such as the 'Pre-Retirement Association', and by health professionals. Nurses in the community or the workplace have a particularly important role to play in promoting retirement preparation, but nurses working in hospitals can also make a contribution. A large proportion of people who choose to retire early do so because of ill health, so it is likely that they will have been in hospital prior to leaving their jobs. Preparation for retirement can include providing the person with information and practical advice about such topics as finance, health and hobbies. It is also important to encourage the person to discuss his own feelings about retirement and to begin to formulate plans. There is some evidence to suggest that the people who adjust best are those who manage to maintain a reasonable amount of continuity between their life before retirement and their life afterwards (Livson, 1962). Thus, it can be helpful to encourage people to develop plans on the basis of their existing interests. It is also important to help people think about the practical implications of their retirement plans. For example, some people decide to retire to distant seaside resorts without considering the fact that they will be moving away from their friends and relatives, and this can lead to problems of social isolation.

Retirement preparation is important because it encourages positive attitudes towards retirement and old age. We prepare and plan for things which are about to begin, but not for things which are about to end. By encouraging people to prepare for retirement, the nurse will convey the message that it is important and valuable and that it marks a new beginning rather than just the end of a person's working life.

SUMMARY

Problems are not an inevitable consequence of old age. However, it is important to understand the reasons for the problems which sometimes affect elderly people so that these can be alleviated.

The first part of this chapter gave an account of communication and memory problems which sometimes affect elderly people, and of how elderly people can be helped to compensate for their difficulties.

The chapter's second part described some of the cognitive, affective and behavioural changes which can affect people with senile dementia. Self-care, individualised patient care and good communication can all make an important contribution to the care of such patients. Reality orientation is an example of an approach which aims to improve communication between people with dementia and their carers.

The final part of the chapter dealt with ways in which elderly people react to the changes in circumstance brought about by admission to an institution and by retirement. There are many ways in which the negative effects of these changes can be reduced or avoided.

It is important to remember that the various problems discussed in this chapter do not affect all elderly people. Furthermore, when problems do occur, there will usually be something that can be done to help the elderly person to cope. The positive aspects of old age such as freedom from the constraints of work must be remembered: old age can be fun, and the nurse can help to make it so.

References

Adams J (1986) Reality orientation: a nursing approach. *Geriatric Nursing*, **6**: 21–23.

Armstrong-Esther C A and Browne K D (1986) The influence of elderly patients' mental impairment on nurse–patient interaction. *Journal of Advanced Nursing*, **11**: 379–387.

Atchley R C (1976) *The Sociology of Retirement*. New York: Schenkman.

Begert L and Jacobsson E (1976) Training of reality orientation with a group of patients with senile dementia. *Scandinavian Journal of Behaviour Therapy*, **5**: 191–200.

Bergman M (1971) Hearing and aging. *Audiology*, **10**: 164–171.

Beveridge W E (1980) Retirement and life significance. *Human Relations*, **33**: 69–78

Botwinick J (1978) *Aging and Behavior*, 2nd edn. New York: Springer.

Burton M (1982) Reality orientation for the elderly: a critique. *Journal of Advanced Nursing*, **7**: 427–433.

Cohen G (1979) Language comprehension in old age. *Cognitive Psychology*, **11**: 412–429.

Corso J F (1977) Auditory perception and communication. In: *Handbook of the Psychology of Aging*, eds. Birren J E and Schaie K W. New York: Van Nostrand Reinhold.

Craik F I M (1977) Age differences in human memory. In: *Handbook of the Psychology of Aging*, eds. Birren J E and Schaie KW. New York: Van Nostrand Reinhold.

Cumming E M and Henry W (1961) *Growing Old*. New York: Basic Books.

Friedmann E A and Orbach H L (1974) Adjustment to retirement. In: *American Handbook of Psychiatry*, ed. Arieti S, vol. 1. New York: Basic Books.

Gilleard C J (1984) *Living with Dementia*. London: Croom Helm.

Gustafsson R (1976) Milieu therapy in a ward for patients with senile dementia. *Scandinavian Journal of Behaviour Therapy*, **5**: 27–39.

Holden U P and Woods R T (1982) *Reality Orientation*. Edinburgh: Churchill Livingstone.

Kausler D H (1982) *Experimental Psychology and Human Aging*. New York: John Wiley.

Kay D W and Bergmann K (1980) Epidemiology of mental disorders amongst the aged in the community. In: *Handbook of Mental Health and Aging*, eds. Birren J E and Sloane R B. Englewood Cliffs, New Jersey: Prentice-Hall.

Langer E J and Rodin J (1976) The effects of choice and enhanced personal responsibility for the aged: a field experiment in an institutional setting. *Journal of Personality and Social Psychology*, **34**: 191–198.

Leech S and Witte K L (1971) Paired-associate learning in elderly adults as related to pacing and incentive conditions. *Developmental Psychology*, **5**: 180.

Lipman A, Slater R and Harris H (1979) The quality of verbal interaction in homes for old people. *Gerontology*, **25**: 275–284.

Livson F (1962) Adjustment to retirement. In: *Aging and Personality*, eds. Reichard S, Livson F and Peterson P C. New York: John Wiley.

MacDonald M L and Settin J M (1978) Reality orientation versus sheltered workshops as treatment for institutionalised aging. *Journal of Gerontology*, **33**: 416–421.

Neugarten B L (1977) Personality and aging. In: *Handbook of the Psychology of Aging*, eds. Birren J E and Schaie K W. New York: Van Nostrand Reinhold.

Orem D E (1980) *Nursing: Concepts of Practice*. London: McGraw Hill.

Parker S (1982) *Work and Retirement*. London: George Allen & Unwin.

Perlmutter M and List J A (1982) Learning in later adulthood. In: *Review of Human Development*, eds. Field T M, Huston A, Quay H C, Troll L and Finley G E. New York: John Wiley.

Peterson R F, Knapp T J, Rosen J C and Pither B F (1977) The effects of furniture arrangement on the behaviour of geriatric patients. *Behaviour Therapy*, **8**: 464–467.

Rabbitt P M A (1981) Talking to the old. *New Society*, **55**: 140–141.

Reifler B V, Larson E and Hanley R S (1982) Co-existence of cognitive impairment and depression in geriatric outpatients. *American Journal of Psychiatry*, **139**: 623–626.

Rhee H A (1974) *Human Ageing and Retirement*. Geneva: International Social Security Association.

Ross E (1968) Effects of challenging and supportive instructions on verbal learning in older persons. *Journal of Educational Psychology*, **59**: 261–266.

Sandman P O, Norberg A, Adolfsson R, Axelsson K and Hedly V (1986) Morning care of patients with Alzheimer-type dementia. A theoretical model based on direct observations. *Journal of Advanced Nursing*, **11**: 369–378.

6
Caring for Children

In the Middle Ages, children were treated as if they were little adults: they were expected to dress like adults, work like adults and generally behave like adults. Nowadays, it is widely recognised that children differ from adults in a number of important ways, such as their ability to communicate, their ability to understand events, their emotional reactions, and their behaviour. On the other hand, research carried out during the past 20 years has shown that in some respects children are very competent and are not too different from adults.

This chapter describes some of the differences and similarities between children and adults which have important implications for nursing care. Even if a nurse is not working on a children's ward, she is likely to be involved in caring for children, since nursing care should be given to the whole family and not just to the patient. Conversely, if the patient is a child, care should be given to the parents as well.

This chapter is divided into four sections:

1. Newborn babies
2. Parent–child relationships
3. Communicating with children
4. Children's understanding of illness

The aim of the chapter is to improve understanding of some of the abilities and needs which children have at particular ages. However, it is important to remember that children, like adults, are all different and develop at different rates. Thus, the ages given for developmental changes are approximate and are likely to vary according to the individual child.

NEWBORN BABIES

Newborn babies are, in some respects, helpless. They need to be fed, changed and carried around, and they spend much of their time sleeping. Thus, it may seem tempting to conclude that it is pointless providing newborns with anything other than physical care, and that newborns are not yet individuals in their own right. However, research has shown that many human abilities are present during the first few weeks of life and that newborns are not all alike: they are remarkably competent human beings and are individuals right from the start of their lives. Consequently, newborns deserve more than basic physical care.

Abilities of newborns

Even in the first few weeks of life, babies possess a wide range of abilities. For example, they are able to suck, to move their heads and limbs and to learn (Bower, 1979). They are also able to feel pain (Macfarlane, 1977). One of the most impressive aspects of newborns' ability is their perceptual ability, that is their ability to perceive their surroundings through the senses of sight, hearing, smell, taste and touch.

Research has shown that immediately after birth babies are able to hear and will turn their eyes in the direction of a sound (Wertheimer, 1961). Also, babies of a few days old can see simple patterns and shapes (Slater, Morison and Rose, 1983), and show a preference for real three-dimensional objects rather than two-dimensional pictures (Slater, Rose and Morison, 1984).

Newborn babies can use their perceptual abilities as a way of starting to get to know people, such as their parents. For instance, six-day-old breast-fed babies are able to recognise the smell of their own mother's breast-pad (Macfarlane, 1977) and, by the age of two weeks babies can usually recognise their mother's face and voice (Carpenter, 1974).

There are, however, limitations to newborns' perceptual abilities. For instance, they cannot see fine details (because their visual acuity is limited), and they are only able to focus their eyes on objects which are about nine inches away from them. (Interestingly, during breast-feeding, the mother's face is usually about nine inches away from the baby's eyes.) Thus, if the nurse wants to give a young infant something to look at, she should choose patterns which are reasonably large and bold with clear contrasts. Also, an object being shown to a newborn should be placed about nine inches away from his eyes. The object can be moved sideways since newborns can follow moving objects with their eyes although their eye and head movements are rather jerky.

Newborn babies are not simply awake or asleep, but can be in a variety of different states of alertness (Macfarlane, 1977):

1. Deep sleep, with regular breathing

2. Light sleep, with irregular breathing and occasional restlessness

3. Drowsiness

4. Awake, eyes open, but quiet rather than excited

5. Awake, eyes open, but moving actively

6. Crying

Not surprisingly, babies are most likely to demonstrate their perceptual abilities when they are in state 4, that is, when they are alert but quiet. During the first week of life, most babies are in state 4 for only about 11 per cent of the time (Wolff, 1963). A baby is more likely to become quiet and alert when he is being held upright or when he is lying with his head propped up, than when he is lying flat on his back.

Communicating with parents about their newborn's abilities

Research into newborn's abilities has important implications for the way babies and their parents should be cared for in maternity wards and by nurses working in the community. Parents have long suspected that from a very early age their babies can see them, hear them and recognise them. Most parents enjoy showing things to and talking to their newborns, but they may feel embarrassed about doing so, since myths still survive about newborns being effectively blind and deaf. Nurses can help to dispel such myths by talking to the baby and by telling parents about their baby's abilities so that they can be reassured that it is indeed sensible to interact with a young baby.

● Mrs Thomson recently gave birth to her first child, Robert. While she is feeding and changing Robert, Mrs Thomson chats to him and smiles at him. One day soon after the birth, Mrs Thomson's father came to visit and, when he saw Mrs Thomson talking to Robert, said, 'You're wasting your time, dear. He's much too young to be able to see or hear anything'. After that, Mrs Thomson felt embarrassed about talking to Robert, especially if there was anyone else present. A nurse in the maternity ward then told Mrs Thomson about some of the abilities which newborn babies have. Mrs Thomson felt very pleased and replied, 'Now I can talk to him without feeling stupid'.

An interesting study by Myers (1982) indicates that parents are likely to benefit from being shown what their baby's abilities are. Parents were given demonstrations of their two- to four-day-old infants' abilities. Four weeks later, these parents were compared to other parents who had not received demonstrations, and were found to be:

● More knowledgeable about their baby's behaviour
● Slightly more self-confident in handling their baby
● Slightly more satisfied with their baby

Myers also found that the fathers who received the demonstrations became more involved in care-taking activities (such as changing and bathing the baby) than those who did not. This implies that showing fathers that their babies have interesting human characteristics is likely to increase their involvement with the baby.

When the nurse wants to demonstrate a newborn's abilities to his parents, she should try to choose a time when the baby is in the alert, quiet state (see above). An alternative way of informing parents about a baby's abilities is to show them a film or video, such as 'Getting to know each other' (distributed by Farley Health Products) or 'Amazing newborn' (distributed by Concord Films Council). Such films can be shown either in antenatal clinics or while a mother is in hospital after her baby's birth.

When communicating with parents it is important to stress that every baby is unique. Babies differ not only in terms of the rate at which they develop but also in terms of the amount of time which they spend in each of the different states of alterness. Furthermore, some are more responsive than others to external stimuli such as sounds (Birns, 1965). For these reasons, the nurse must be careful not to give parents the impression that there is something wrong if their baby does not demonstrate a particular ability at exactly the same age as the baby featured in the film.

Particular sensitivity is required when communicating with parents whose baby has been born prematurely. Premature babies may show certain abilities later than full-term babies (Friedman, Jacobs and Werthmann, 1981) which is not surprising since, so far as time from conception is concerned, premature babies are 'younger' than full-term babies born on the same day. On the other hand, premature babies do possess a considerable range of abilities, and it is important to help parents appreciate what their baby can do rather than focusing on what he cannot yet do.

Stern and Hildebrandt (1986) investigated the effects of labelling babies as 'premature'. They observed women interacting with babies whom they had not previously met, all of whom were full-term. However, some of the women were told that the baby they were looking after was premature, while others were correctly told that he was full-term. The women who believed they were interacting with a premature baby had less positive attitudes towards the baby (for example, liked him less) and touched him less than the other women did. These results suggest that the label 'premature' may have negative effects on parents' behaviour towards their baby. Parents of babies born prematurely will, of course, know that their baby is premature. Nevertheless, a nurse can help to encourage positive attitudes towards the baby by emphasising his individuality and his abilities, and by avoiding comments like, 'You can't expect much from a premature baby'.

With both premature and full-term babies, the aim should be to encourage parents to enjoy observing and interacting with their baby in a natural way. Carers should try to respect the newborn's individuality and be responsive to his needs. Most mothers are naturally very good at this and can readily adapt to their baby's interactional style (Schaffer, 1977). However, in cases where parents (or nurses) are uncertain about how to behave towards a young baby, a useful strategy is for them to match their behaviour to the baby's state of alertness (see above). For example, a baby who is awake and quiet (state 4) can be entertained by interesting sights and sounds, whereas a baby who is drowsy (state 3) should not be perceptually stimulated. Babies, like adults (see chapter 2), will often avoid eye contact when they want to end an interaction. When a baby is awake and active (state 5) the carer could try interacting with him by copying his level of activity and imitating some of his behaviours, such as his gestures and facial expressions.

PARENT-CHILD RELATIONSHIPS

Understanding relationships between children and their parents will enable the nurse to provide better nursing care. For example, such understanding should make it easier for her to appreciate the importance of:

- Minimising the number of separations between children and parents
- Helping children and parents to cope when separations do occur
- Involving parents in the care of their children
- Providing emotional support for parents whose children are ill
- Providing emotional support for children whose parents are ill
- Being prepared to learn from parents about how best she can help care for their child

In this section, the development of parent-child relationships is considered, first from the point of view of the parents and then from the point of view of the child. Finally, these two perspectives are combined in an account of the nature of parent–child interaction.

The parents' perspective

The term 'maternal bonding' refers to the development of a loving relationship between a mother and her baby. Three main questions arise regarding bonding:

1. When does it happen?
2. How does it happen?
3. Who is involved in it?

Each of these questions has received two conflicting answers, a 'simple' answer and a 'complex' answer. Although the simple view of bonding has had a considerable impact on nursing practice, it is actually an over-simplification and so carries misleading implications (Sluckin, Herbert and Sluckin, 1983).

The simple view

According to this view, bonding occurs rapidly soon after birth (Klaus et al, 1972). Indeed, the first few hours or days of life are regarded as a sensitive period for bonding, which implies that there is something special about this very early period and that, if bonding does not occur at this time, later difficulties in the mother-child relationship are likely. In answer to 'How does it happen?' it has been argued that skin-to-skin contact between mother and baby during this sensitive period plays a crucial role in the bonding process, and that the mother's hormone levels immediately after birth make her particularly receptive to the development of a strong emotional tie with her baby. This explanation in terms of hormones implies the simple answer to the 'Who' question: that bonding is unique to the biological mother.

The complex view

According to this view, a mother's bond with her child develops gradually over a period of months or even years, and the period immediately after birth does not have overriding significance. Also, the time at which a mother begins to develop a bond with her baby varies from mother to mother, as Macfarlane (1977) found in a study where he asked mothers when they had started to feel love towards their first-born babies. While some mothers said it was at birth, others said it was during pregnancy, during the first week after birth or, for some, later than the first week after birth.

The complex answer to the 'How' question is that bonds develop as a result of parents' experiences of interacting with their children. In other words, parents gradually 'get to know' their children through communicating with them, thinking about them, playing with them, holding them and catering for their physical needs.

The complex view recognises that bonding is not unique to the biological mother: fathers and adoptive parents can also develop strong bonds with their children (Parke, 1981; Tizard, 1977). Furthermore, the baby makes an important contribution to the development of a bond, since the way parents interact with their baby is affected by characteristics of the individual baby (Schaffer, 1977).

Which view is correct?

Research provides more support for the complex than for the simple view of bonding (Sluckin, Herbert and Sluckin, 1983). Thus, the quality of a parent–child relationship depends on the quality of parent–child interaction, which in turn can be influenced by a whole multitude of factors, such as the characteristics of the parents, of the child and of the environment in which the child is brought up. This does not mean that skin-to-skin contact immediately after birth is totally unimportant: it is one form of parent–child interaction, so can contribute to the development of a mother–child relationship. However, although this very early interaction is often extremely rewarding and poignant for the mother, research has shown that its long-term effect on the mother's relationship with her child does not outweigh the effects of other, later experiences of parent–child interaction.

Implications for nursing

Although the simple view of bonding has had a considerable impact on nursing, it has negative as well as positive implications. By, instead, basing nursing care on the complex view of bonding, the negative consequences can be reduced while the positive consequences of the simple view are retained.

On the positive side, the simple view of bonding has encouraged the practice of allowing mothers to have physical contact with their babies immediately after birth, and has reduced the extent to which mothers and babies are likely to be separated from one another during their stay in hospital. Since the complex view of bonding stresses the importance of all parent–child interactions, it also implies that mothers should be given every opportunity to be with their newborn babies so that they can start getting to know each other. Indeed, the same applies to fathers.

Negative consequences of the simple view of bonding are likely to arise in cases where immediate skin-to-skin contact is either not possible, or not desired by the mother. For example, if a baby is born prematurely, he may well have to be placed in an incubator immediately after birth and, as a result, opportunities for early physical contact between mother and baby are likely to be limited or absent. The admission of a newborn baby to a neonatal unit is extremely traumatic for his parents. Not only will they feel anxious about the possibility of him dying or being permanently disabled, but they are also likely to experience feelings of guilt and to think that they may have been responsible for their baby's condition (Richards, 1978). Belief in the simple view of bonding can add to these parents' feelings of anxiety and guilt, since it implies that the mother and child have missed out on a crucial early experience and that this will permanently hamper their relationship. Such a belief could well become a self-fulfilling prophecy, in that the feelings of guilt and anxiety may themselves interfere with the development of a good parent–child relationship.

In contrast, the complex view of bonding offers hope in such circumstances, since it indicates that future experiences can compensate for the 'missed' early experience. Many parents will have read or heard about the simple view of bonding, so it is important to reassure them that parent–child relationships can be developed gradually and at any time. They should not be allowed to feel that they have missed their only opportunity of developing a good relationship with their child.

On the other hand, it is important to recognise that there are several factors, other than lack of skin-to-skin contact, which may interfere with parents' ability to form relationships with babies who are admitted to a neonatal unit. Parents' feelings of guilt and anxiety have already been mentioned. In addition, premature babies tend to be less physically attractive than full-term babies, and the 'beautiful is good' bias may influence parents' perception of their baby (see chapter 4). Not surprisingly, ill babies are typically more difficult to handle than healthy babies; for instance, they may cry more and be more difficult to soothe. Sometimes parents report that they feel as if the baby belongs to the staff rather than to them (Richards, 1978).

For all these reasons, it is important to give good psychological care to the parents of babies in neonatal units. In particular, parents should be given opportunities to talk to the nurses about their feelings of anxiety and guilt. The nurse should encourage parents to express their feelings by asking exploratory questions and by responding in a non-judgmental way if they express guilt or anxiety (see chapter 2). Parents should also be offered as many opportunities as possible of getting to know their baby and of contributing to his care. For example, they could be encouraged to touch, stroke and talk to their baby. If the baby is called by the name his parents have chosen, and dressed in clothes which his parents have selected, the parents will be helped to feel that the baby is theirs.

Similar arguments apply to cases where the mother feels unable or unwilling to engage in skin-to-skin contact with her infant immediately after birth. For instance, if the baby has been delivered by caesarian section or if the birth has been difficult, the mother may feel too ill or exhausted to be interested in 'bonding' with her baby. These mothers should not be made to feel guilty, and should be reassured that there will be plenty of time to get to know the baby when they feel ready. A mother who has abdominal wounds may find it difficult to feed and cuddle her baby, but a nurse may sometimes be able to suggest ways round such problems. For example, the mother may find it easier to breast feed lying down rather than in the conventional sitting position.

While it is important to provide the opportunity for contact from the moment of birth, it is equally important to allow parents to choose when to interact with their baby. In other words, the nurse should, by basing her care on the family's needs, provide individualised rather than task-oriented care.

The child's perspective

At about the age of seven months, children usually begin to demonstrate that they have formed strong attachments to particular people.

Early research suggested that young children develop a strong attachment to only one person, and that this unique, exclusive bond with a 'mother-figure' is essential to the child's psychological well-being (Bowlby, 1958). However, further research has shown that, by the age of 18 months, most children have developed strong relationships with more than one person (Schaffer and Emerson, 1964). Many children have strong bonds with both their parents, and some children also have bonds with siblings, grandparents, other relatives or neighbours. Furthermore, the quality of a child's relationships does not seem to be diluted by increased quantity. For example, a child who has attachments to his mother, his father and his sister can have just as deep a relationship with his mother as can a child who is attached only to his mother.

Children's strongest attachments are not always to the people who are most involved in providing them with physical care; i.e. children's relationships are not simply based on 'cupboard love'. Although psychologists do not yet fully understand how relationships develop, there is considerable evidence that children tend to develop attachments to people who interact with them regularly, and that children probably develop their strongest attachments to those people with whom they have the most satisfying interactions (Schaffer, 1977). Of course, this raises the issue of what makes for a satisfying interaction. Schaffer proposes that some of the important qualities are sensitivity, responsiveness and emotional involvement.

Separation

From about the age of seven or eight months until about four years old, many children will show distress if they are separated from someone with whom they have a strong attachment. This is known as *separation anxiety*. Separation anxiety is usually at its peak between the ages of about 14 and 18 months, after which it begins to decline. At approximately the same age as they show separation anxiety, children may also show *stranger fear*, that is, they will become upset by the presence of an unfamiliar person even if their mother (or another familiar person) is with them. Separation anxiety and stranger fear both involve the child demonstrating a strong preference for a particular person's company, so the emergence of these reactions provides evidence that the child has developed an attachment to a specific person.

A child who is showing separation anxiety will typically respond to the departure of a loved one by crying and screaming. If the separation is prolonged, the *protest* phase may give way to the *despair* phase, during which the child will quieten down but will become miserable and apathetic. Finally, the child may enter the *detachment* phase: he seems to be contented but when his parents return he is likely to show no interest in them (Bowlby, 1973).

Although some children do not show separation anxiety, others show extreme distress when separated from their parents. When children are ill, tired or frightened, they are particularly likely to want to stay close to their parents, so there is an increased risk of them showing separation anxiety. For these reasons when young children are admitted to hospital every effort should be made to avoid separating them from their parents. Anyone who doubts the importance of this advice should watch some of the films produced by James and Joyce Robertson, which provide a very powerful portrayal of the severity of some young children's reactions to separation (e.g. Robertson and Robertson, 1968).

Older children are less likely than younger children to show obvious signs of distress in response to separation. Nevertheless, older children are also likely to benefit from their parents' company while in hospital. Ross and Ross (1984) asked five- to 12-year-olds what would have helped them most when they were experiencing the worst pain they had ever had. Almost without exception, the children replied that having their parents present would be the thing which would help most.

Avoiding separations between children and their parents can contribute not only to children's psychological well-being but also to their physical well-being. For example, Brain and Maclay (1968) found that children whose mothers stayed in hospital with them were less likely to develop infections after tonsillectomy than were children admitted without their mothers. This is an interesting and important finding, since one reason which hospital staff sometimes give for restricting parents' contact with their children is the risk of infection.

In recent years, there has been an increasing awareness of the importance of keeping separation to a minimum when children are admitted to hospital. As a result, more and more children's wards have introduced arrangements for flexible visiting and for parents to stay overnight. However, facilities and policies differ widely from one hospital to another and in some cases are still far from ideal (Consumers' Association, 1980; Stenbak, 1986). Also, several authors have noted that what actually happens on a particular ward does not always coincide with either the expressed hospital policy or the available facilities (Poster, 1983; Rodin, 1983; Crawford-Blitzer et al, 1983; Muller, Harris and Wattley, 1986). For example, sometimes the policy is to allow unrestricted visiting, but the ward staff introduce restrictions by asking parents to leave at particular times, or by making it obvious to parents that they are 'in the way'. In other cases, parents do not make use of the available facilities because they are unaware of the importance of their presence to the child. The nurse can play a very important role by ensuring that parents are aware of the contribution they can make, and by providing a welcoming atmosphere so that parents will be encouraged to spend time in the hospital.

Although it is important to give parents the opportunity to become involved in caring for their child in hospital, nurses should also be involved in caring for both the child and for the family. Looking after an ill child is a stressful experience, and the parents' feelings of stress may increase if they feel that the nurses are leaving them to cope entirely on their own. A nurse can offer valuable support by showing her willingness to share responsibility for the child's care with the parents, and by taking time to develop a relationship with both parents and child. If a nurse talks to and plays with the child while the parents are present, this will probably help the child to regard the nurse as a friend who can provide comfort should the parents have to leave. The needs of all members of the family (and particularly of any siblings of the ill child) should be considered. Sometimes the parents will devote so much of their time and attention to the child who is ill that his siblings feel neglected. A nurse can tactfully offer to sit with the ill child so that the parents can go and spend some time with their other children. Also, when the siblings are in the ward, a nurse could give them some of her attention and encourage them to become involved in the ward's play activities.

Separations between children and their parents cannot always be completely avoided during hospitalisation. Research into children's reactions to separation (summarised in Rutter, 1981) suggests that there are a number of ways in which children can be helped to cope with separation.

1. Children typically become less upset by separations if they are able to keep to a familiar routine. Therefore, when a child is admitted, the nursing staff should enquire about his usual routine, for example, how he asks to go to the toilet, whether he has a special bed-time ritual, what his favourite toys are called and which are his favourite television programmes.

2. Most children have relationships with more than one person. This means that separation from one particular person, for example the mother, can often be made less distressing if another familiar person can be present instead. It is helpful to

discuss this with the parents before the child is admitted so that they have more time to arrange a visiting rota, and also so that they can make appropriate arrangements for the care of other children in the family. A further consequence of children having multiple attachments is that they may well miss people other than their parents while they are in hospital. For example, they may miss their brothers, sisters, friends and pets. Thus, it is a good idea to find out who a child would like to see, and to try to encourage visits from these people. This is particularly important if the child's stay in hospital is to be a long one.

3. Children find separations more distressing when they are in an unfamiliar environment than when they are in a familiar one. Hospital environments are, of course, very different from the home environments which children are used to. However, the strangeness of the hospital can be reduced somewhat by encouraging children to visit it with their parents before admission, and by ensuring that, on admission, children are shown around and given the opportunity to explore their new surroundings while their parents are still with them. It is important to make the ward as homely as possible. For example, there should be colourful pictures on the walls, play materials and somewhere for the children to play together. Children should be encouraged to bring a selection of their belongings into hospital, as this can help them to feel more at home. It is advisable to attach a name band to Teddy to make sure that he does not get lost. Sometimes young children are particularly attached to a specific soft toy or other 'comfort' object, such as a blanket. Since these treasured possessions tend to go everywhere with the child, they often become very tattered. Therefore, it may be necessary to reassure embarrassed parents that these precious objects are welcome in hospital. Providing comfort for the child is far more important than ensuring that everything in the ward looks new and shiny.

4. If children are given the opportunity to form new relationships, they will usually find it easier to cope with a separation. For example, getting to know one of the nurses or one of the other children in the ward is likely to reduce their feelings of distress about being away from their parents. However, children can develop relationships only if they have the chance to spend a reasonable amount of time interacting with a particular person. This is a strong argument for assigning particular nurses to particular children (that is, using individualised or primary care) rather than having a task-oriented system of care. The nurse ought also to spend time talking to and playing with the children, and encouraging them to play with one another.

5. Separation anxiety declines as children grow older. One of the most probable reasons for this is that older children are more able to understand explanations about parents' departures and reassurances about their return. It is important to ensure that children are actually given such explanations and reassurances. Like adults, children will probably feel more secure and more 'in control' when they are able to see events as being predictable and explicable rather than haphazard. Even young children should be given explanations, but extra care should be taken to express these simply. In particular, it is important to realise that young children do not usually understand descriptions of time in the same way as adults do, and that time seems to pass more slowly for children than for older people. If, for example,

the nurse tells a young child whose mother is going to be away for several hours that, 'Mummy won't be long', he may well interpret this as meaning that Mummy will be back in a few minutes, just as she is when she pops into the kitchen to boil the kettle. It is generally better to avoid phrases like 'long' and 'soon', and to refer instead to specific events in the child's daily routine, for example, 'Mummy will come back after you have had your lunch' (provided, of course, that the nurse knows this will happen).

Although this section has focused on ways of helping children to cope with separation, the points which have been made also apply in a general form to situations where separation does not occur. Thus, when caring for children in hospital, it is important to try to find out about their usual routines, to encourage visitors, to make the ward homely, to help children to develop relationships with staff and patients and to provide explanations. This will help both the children and their parents to cope successfully with the experience of being in hospital.

Parent–child interaction

Interaction and communication play a central role in the development of parent–child relationships. Long before children begin to talk, they are capable of communicating non-verbally with their parents. Research on these early interactions indicates that at a very early stage in the child's life three important characteristics of parent–child relationships begin to develop:
1. Uniqueness
2. Reciprocity
3. Shared feelings

Uniqueness

During the first few months of a baby's life, each mother–infant pair will usually develop a unique interaction pattern, their own special way of responding to one another (Stern, 1977; Trevarthen, 1977).

Reciprocity

Reciprocity occurs when two people respond to one another's behaviour and influence one another. Imitation is one of the earliest forms of reciprocity in the mother–infant interaction, and can occur as early as the first week of a baby's life (Meltzoff and Moore, 1977). For example, a baby will sometimes imitate his mother when she opens her mouth, sticks out her tongue or moves her fingers. In such cases, the baby's behaviour is being influenced by that of his mother. On other occasions, mothers will imitate aspects of their babies' behaviour, such as their facial expression (Trevarthen, 1977). However, early mother–infant interaction is certainly not restricted to imitation; there are a wide variety of ways in which mothers and infants can respond to each other's behaviour.

In most mother–infant interactions, the mother's and infant's contributions fit together in terms of their timing. Trevarthen (1977) observed that when two-month-old infants are interacting with their mothers, the mothers' and the infants' actions typically alternate in a regular manner: the baby does something, then the mother reacts, then the baby does something else, and so on. It is as if they are having a conversation in that they take turns at being the active participant. The baby's actions can include head and limb movements, smiling and other facial expressions, lip and tongue movements, and vocalisations (such as coos and gurgles). The mother may produce similar actions, and in addition she is likely to speak to the baby.

Shared feelings

The mother's and infant's actions usually also fit together in terms of their emotional quality. Sometimes, the exchange may be excited and animated, whereas at other times it may be calm and subdued (Stern, 1977). Through their interaction, the mother and infant are sharing different types of emotional experiences.

The characteristics of uniqueness, reciprocity and shared feelings all contribute to the sense of closeness and mutal understanding which typify most parent-child relationships. This has several important implications for nursing.

1. Because of the reciprocity and the ability to share feelings which characterise parent–child relationships, parents are likely to feel anxiety and distress when their children are anxious, distressed or in pain. It it therefore important to provide parents with emotional support in such situations. For example, parents should be given opportunities to talk about their feelings and, when they do so, they should be offered acceptance and realistic reassurance. A similar point applies when it is the parent who is ill. In such cases, emotional support should be given to the children.

2. Providing support for the parents of an ill child can contribute to the psychological care of the child, again because of the shared feelings and reciprocity of parent–child relationships. Parents are in a strong position to provide emotional support for their child, so long as they themselves feel reassured.

3. Parents can provide invaluable advice about how best to care for their child. This is because they will usually have accumulated considerable knowledge about their child, for example knowledge about how the child is likely to react, how he might feel and what he is capable of doing and of understanding. Similarly, the nurse can learn a great deal about how to behave towards a particular child by watching his parents interacting with him.

4. Parents should be encouraged to become involved in caring for their child while he is in hospital. Parents and children are used to responding to one another, so it is likely to be disconcerting for both parent and child if the parent is left sitting passively while the nurses rush around doing everything for the child. It is always important to involve relatives in the patient's care, but this is even more important when the patient is a child. It must be remembered that, while the nurse often knows more about the child's medical condition than do the parents, the parents will certainly know more than the nurse about their child. The nurse's aim should be to work with the parents as a team.

Older children

Although the research findings reported in this section relate to very young children, the nursing implications outlined are relevant to children of all ages.

The nature of a parent–child relationship certainly changes with age, but it does not usually weaken. For instance, children over the age of four years are generally better than younger children at coping with separations from their parents, but this does not mean that a five-year-old's relationship with his parents is less strong than that of a two-year-old. In one sense, the five-year-old's relationship is stronger in that it is more secure: the child is now more confident that the relationship will endure despite separations. One probable reason for this change in the parent–child relationship is that the nature of the interaction changes as the child grows older. In particular, once the child acquires language and is no longer restricted to non-verbal communication, interactions can move beyond the 'here and now'. With the development of verbal communication, it becomes increasingly possible to communicate about absent people and about future points in time. It also becomes increasingly possible to communicate *with* absent people, for example, by means of the telephone and letters. Thus, as interactions move beyond the immediate context by becoming more verbal, parent–child relationships can also move beyond the 'here and now' by becoming less dependent on physical contact and close proximity.

COMMUNICATING WITH CHILDREN

The previous section showed that children are able to communicate non-verbally long before they learn to talk. This section focuses mainly on the development of verbal communication, and its aim is to provide an overview of children's language abilities so that the nurse will be better able to:

- Understand what children are trying to say to her
- Help children understand what she is saying

There are two main reasons why successful communication with children is important. First, communication plays a major role in the development of relationships so communicating with a child will help the nurse to establish a relationship with him. Second, as with adult patients, communication is likely to contribute to a child's sense of control over his environment. For example, if the child can understand the nurse she will be able to give him information and explanations about what is going to happen. And if she can understand what the child is saying, she will be in a better position to assess his needs and wishes.

The first words

Most children begin to produce recognisable words somewhere between the ages of 10 and 15 months. However, children often do not pronounce these early words in the same way as an adult would. Most early words consist of a consonant followed by a vowel (e.g. 'ma') or of a duplication of this pattern (e.g. 'mama'). Young children have difficulty producing some sounds (e.g. 's' and 'f') and they also have difficulty producing consonant clusters (such as the 'lk' in 'milk'). Some children have problems with pronunciation up until the age of four or five years.

Various strategies are used by young children to simplify the pronunciation of words, and different children use different strategies. Consequently, while a child's first words may be recognisable to his parents (and to other familiar people), they may not be recognisable to a stranger. This means that when communicating with young children it is often useful to involve the child's parents (or siblings) in the conversation to explain what the child is saying. On the other hand, the nurse must not just take the easy way out and talk to the parents as if the child was not present. If the nurse talks to the child, she will become familiar with his pronunciation.

Up until the age of about 18 months to two years, children's speech consists only of single words; they are not yet able to combine words to form sentences. However, some researchers (e.g. Bloom, 1973) have argued that young children use a single word to convey a meaning similar to that which an adult would convey using a full sentence. For example, a young child may use the word 'Dada' to mean 'Look, there's Daddy', or 'Where is Daddy?', or 'I want Daddy', or 'This is Daddy's chair'. The person who is listening to the child has to work out which meaning is appropriate on the basis of the child's intonation and the context in which the word is produced. Of course, we cannot be certain that young children really do intend to convey so much information with a single word but, on the other hand, it is certainly the case that most parents try to read as much meaning as possible into their young children's single words. This general principle, that young children do have more to say than is immediately apparent and that it is worth while trying hard to understand them, is a very useful one to follow when communicating with young children.

The first sentences

When children do start combining words (usually between 18 months and two years of age), they are only able to produce combinations of two words, such as 'Dada car'. As with children's single-word speech, it is necessary to look for cues in the context to work out what the child's two-word combinations are likely to mean. The two-word stage usually last for about six months. During the next two or three years, children learn to produce sentences which are longer and more grammatically complex. By the time children are about four or five years old, their sentences are usually quite similar to those of adults. A five-year-old's speech is still likely to contain a few grammatical errors, and there are some grammatical structures which are not acquired until after the age of five. The pre-school period is, however, the time when children's language ability is developing most rapidly and dramatically.

Meaning

Young children's ideas about what words mean sometimes differ from those of adults. Even if a child is using a particular word, it should not automatically be assumed that he understands its meaning in exactly the same way as would an adult. For example, children sometimes use words in ways which are too general from the point of view of adult usage. Such errors are known as *overextensions*. Examples of overextensions would be calling all animals 'doggies' or calling all men 'Daddy' (much to the

embarrassment of the child's mother). The age at which overextensions are particularly likely to occur is between about one year and two years six months, but they can
also occur at later stages. Sometimes, children make other types of errors, such as
giving a particular word a meaning which is too narrow.

There are two main ways in which one can find out about an individual child's
understanding of word meaning. These are:

1. By listening carefully to how the child uses a particular word on a variety of
   occasions
2. By talking to the child's parents about what they think the child understands by
   particular words which are important to the child's care.

Understanding language: the role of context

It is frequently observed, by both parents and researchers, that young children seem
to be better at understanding language than at using it. However, it is very difficult
to be sure how much of children's understanding of a conversation is actually based
on their comprehension of language itself. This is because young children often draw
heavily on non-verbal cues when they are trying to make sense of what is being said
(Macnamara, 1977).

Imagine a situation in which a mother holds out a newspaper towards her 18-
month-old son, points in the direction of her husband and says, 'Take the paper to
Daddy, please, Simon'. Simon shows no hesitation in carrying out the action which
his mother has requested. However this does not necessarily mean that Simon has
fully understood what his mother said. He might have been responding to non-verbal
cues, such as his mother's gestures of holding out the newspaper and pointing towards
his father. Alternatively, he might have understood some of the words in his mother's
sentence, such as 'Daddy' and 'Simon', and have worked out the rest from the context.

When communicating with young children, it is very important to provide a
non-verbal context which helps them to understand what is being said, for example,
pointing to objects while talking about them or, if possible, holding the items out to
the children and letting them handle them. Pictures are another very useful way of
providing contextual support: photographs and pictures from books or magazines
can be used, or the nurse can draw her own pictures and encourage the child to do
so too. When explaining a procedure to a child, the nurse should demonstrate what
will happen while describing it. Sometimes dolls, puppets or other toys can be used
to act out a procedure or situation with the child.

Research has shown that, if there is a conflict between verbal and non-verbal
information, young children tend to respond to the message which is being conveyed
non-verbally (Macnamara, 1977). Thus, the nurse should try to ensure that her
non-verbal message does not conflict with her verbal message. For example, there is
no point in the nurse telling a child that everything will be all right if her facial
expression is sad and anxious.

Eye contact plays an important role in communiation with children, just as it does
in communication with adults (see chapter 2). In order to establish eye contact with
a young child, the carer needs to bend down or pick the child up so that her eyes are
on the same level as the child's.

Young children are likely to communicate best in contexts where they are talking about familiar things with a familiar adult, and where they feel that they are sharing an activity with the adult rather than being 'tested'. For example, Tizard and Hughes (1984) observed four-year-olds' conversations with their mothers at home and with their teachers at nursery school, and found that the communication abilities which the children demonstrated in the home context were far superior to those which they demonstrated in the nursery school context.

Tizard and Hughes' findings have important implications for nursing contexts. Communication with young children is likely to be more successful in situations which mimic a home environment rather than a school environment. For instance, the nurse should not just rush up to a child, ask a string of questions and then rush away again. She should instead try to become involved with the child (for example, through playing with him) and build up a conversation around what she is doing. The first aim should be to help the child to feel relaxed and to encourage him to talk about whatever he wants. Those things which the nurse wants to talk about should be introduced gradually and casually so that the child does not feel that he is being tested. A useful first step (especially with very shy children) is to begin by observing the child interacting with his parents and then gradually to become involved in the interaction. It is also important to find out as much as possible about each child's background and previous experiences in order to bring these into the conversation as appropriate.

Although creating a 'testing' atmosphere should be avoided, there will, of course, be situations where the nurse needs to check that the child has understood what has been said. Again, it is important to do this in as informal a way as possible. Pre-school children usually enjoy fantasy play in which they talk to cuddly toy animals or puppets, so one way of checking a young child's understanding of an explanation is to ask him to give the explanation to a toy. (This type of technique has been used successfully in several studies of pre-school children's language, e.g. Donaldson, 1978; Donaldson, 1986).

This section has covered some general points about how to communicate with children. These points provide a foundation for the next section, which will focus on the more specific issue of how to communicate with children about illness.

CHILDREN'S UNDERSTANDING OF ILLNESS

From an early age, most children actively seek to make sense of the world around them. They want to know why things happen and if adults do not provide explanations children will often come up with their own. In some cases when children produce their own explanations of illness, the fantasy is worse than the reality. Thus, as soon as a child is able to understand language, he should be given some explanation of his illness and of the treatment he is receiving. Children, like adults, are likely to feel more in control and more able to cope if they are informed of what is happening to them. On the other hand, a young child will obviously be unable to understand a complicated explanation. The starting point for the explanation given to a child should be his own knowledge about illness. This section deals with two main aspects of children's understanding of illness:

1. Children's knowledge of the inside of their bodies
2. Children's understanding of the causes of illness

Preoperative preparation of children and children's understanding of treatment are covered in chapter 7.

Knowledge of the inside of the body

When communicating with children, it is important to remember that they have not had the benefit of reading anatomy and physiology textbooks. Most young children will have received little or no formal instruction about what goes on inside their bodies. This, combined with the fact that the inside of the body cannot be directly observed, means that we should not have high expectations about children's knowledge in this area.

On the other hand, children are not totally ignorant about their 'insides'. When children are asked what is inside their bodies, most of them are able by the age of seven years to name or draw the brain, heart, bones and blood. Older children (10- to 12-year-olds) will usually also mention the stomach and lungs (Porter, 1974; Crider, 1981; Eiser and Patterson, 1983).

Similarly, as children get older they gradually develop a more complex understanding of the functions of different body parts. For example, when children are asked which body parts are involved in the process of eating, six-year-olds mention the mouth and say that food goes into the stomach, although they are unsure about what happens next. Some eight-year-olds know that waste products are excreted and they may mention some of the relevant body parts. Also, some eight-year-olds know that food is circulated around the body, but very few children, even by the age of 12, know that this is achieved through the bloodstream (Eiser and Patterson, 1983).

Since different children are likely to have different amounts and areas of knowledge, it is useful to talk to individual children about their knowledge of their bodies. The nurse can then attempt to build on and extend their existing knowledge in a simple, step-by-step way, and can also try to dispel any frightening misunderstandings which they may have.

● Seven-year-old Edward was extremely anxious and distressed on admission to hospital for a minor operation. Through talking to Edward and encouraging him to talk about his fears, a nurse discovered that Edward was scared about being 'cut' in the operation because another child had told him that all his blood would 'drop out'. The nurse was able to reassure Edward by explaining to him that his blood would clot and that the surgeon would make sure he did not lose it.

It is a good idea to make use of non-verbal communication to help children to understand about the insides of their bodies. For example, when mentioning a particular internal body part, the nurse could simultaneously point to the corresponding part on the outside of the child's body and say something like, 'Your lungs are inside here'. Also, it can be helpful to show children diagrams or models of internal organs, or to make a sketch to illustrate the explanation.

Children's understanding of the causes of illness

In order to understand causes of illness, it is necessary to understand processes which take place inside the body and how these processes interact with various external factors. Thus, children's explanations of illness are likely to be limited by their insecure grasp of what happens inside their bodies. It is also worth remembering that adult lay people too are often at a loss to explain their illnesses (see chapter 3), as sometimes are doctors and nurses.

Research has suggested that different age groups of children have different ideas about how illness is caused. These research findings will be summarised in relation to three age-groups: four- to seven-year-olds, seven- to 11-year-olds, and over 11-year-olds.

Four- to seven-year-olds

The most common explanations of illness given by children in this age group are based on the concept of contagion; that is, children seem to view illness as resulting from mere proximity to particular objects or people (Bibace and Walsh, 1980).

Furthermore, Kister and Patterson (1980) found that four- and five-year-olds tend to overgeneralise the contagion type of explanation, in that they apply it not only to contagious illnesses (such as colds) but also to non-contagious conditions (such as toothache and scraped knees). This finding has important practical implications. First, special effort is likely to be required when explaining non-contagious illness to young children, since they may find such illness harder to understand than contagious illness. Second, young children may become distressed about the risk of catching a non-contagious illness through proximity to someone who has that illness. It is important that the nurse is aware of the possibility of such fears in order to offer appropriate reassurance, for example, a simple explanation of how the particular non-contagious condition is caused.

- Four-year-old Andrew was admitted to hospital for a tonsillectomy. In the next bed to Andrew was an eight-year-old called Stephen who was about to have an appendectomy. Stephen was frequently heard complaining of a 'terribly sore tummy'. Andrew played quite happily during the day, but when it was time to go to bed, he started crying and tried to resist being put into bed. When Andrew's mother eventually succeeded in putting him to bed, he moved right over to the edge of the bed which was furthest away from Stephen and said, 'I don't want to get a sore tummy'. The nurse said to Andrew, 'Stephen has a special kind of sore tummy. When Stephen was born, a bit of his tummy had not been made quite right, so sometimes when Stephen eats, the food gets blocked up and makes his tummy sore. Tomorrow, the doctors are going to mend Stephen's tummy. You won't get Stephen's sore tummy because your tummy doesn't need to be mended. You could go right up to Stephen and touch him, and you still would not get his sore tummy.' Andrew was reassured by this explanation. After a little while, he moved into the middle of his bed and fell asleep.

Some (though by no means all) four- to five-year-olds explain illness as a punishment for their own misbehaviour (Kister and Patterson, 1980) and this can lead to children feeling guilty about being ill. In Kister and Patterson's study, children who had a good understanding of the actual causes of illness were less likely to regard illness as a punishment. This suggests that it might be possible to reduce the risk of children feeling guilty by helping them understand how particular illnesses are caused.

Seven- to eleven-year-olds

By about the age of seven years, children have usually realised that illnesses are not caught simply by being close to someone who is ill. They now believe that for illness to be transmitted there has to be some concrete mechanism of contamination, such as physical contact (Bibace and Walsh, 1980). Thus, a child in this age group may say that one becomes ill by touching someone who is ill. Another common explanation among seven- to 11-year-olds is that illness is caused by germs (Perrin and Gerrity, 1981).

Over eleven-year-olds

By this age, children are becoming aware that illness involves something going wrong inside the body, even though they cannot always supply details about exactly what might go wrong. In explaining illness, 11-year-olds often mention such processes as swallowing and inhaling, by which external causes can influence internal bodily processes (Bibace and Walsh, 1980).

After the age of 11, children's explanations of illness become increasingly complex and sophisticated. For example, children in this oldest age group may describe the cause of an illness in terms of the malfunctioning of specific internal organs or processes, and they may demonstrate an awareness that illness can be influenced by psychological factors, such as thoughts and feelings (Bibace and Walsh, 1980). Also, research by Brewster (1982) has shown that older children usually realise that:

● Different diseases have different causes
● A particular illness can have multiple causes
● Factors external to the body interact with internal factors to cause illness

Thus, older children no longer view their bodies as being passive in relation to illness, but are becoming aware of such concepts as resistance and susceptibility.

Nursing implications

Taken at face value, the research into children's understanding of their bodies and of illness may seem to imply that nurses should restrict their explanations to the level which has been shown to be characteristic of a particular age group. However, this implication is not valid, for two main reasons.

First, the stages which have been described are based on the average answers given by a particular age group. In all the studies there was considerable variation in the level of answer given within each age group: some children gave explanations characteristic of children younger than themselves, while other children gave explanations characteristic of older children. Thus, although the stages outlined are a useful guide to what to expect from children of a particular age, it is important not to take the ages too literally and to remember that each child is an individual. As far as possible, the individual child's understanding of illness should be clarified.

Second, it is possible that the answers which the children gave to the researchers' questions did not represent the limits of their ability to understand illness. Since most young children will not have received much tuition about illness, their answers to researchers' questions may merely reflect what they have had the opportunity to learn. It may well be that they would be capable of understanding more if they were taught in an appropriate way.

Thus, at present, we do not really know how much children of a particular age are capable of understanding about illness. The practical implication of this is that the nurse should:

● Try to establish what the individual child understands about illness
● Gradually introduce more information and more complex explanations

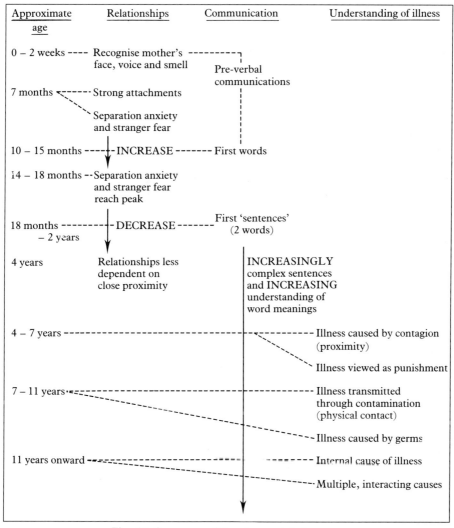

Fig. 6.1 Summary of developmental changes.

- At frequent intervals check whether the child has understood her explanations. More complex explanations should not be provided until it has been established that the child has understood the more basic explanations.

SUMMARY

This chapter has demonstrated the importance of providing psychological care for children and their parents. Even newborn babies are individuals and have basic human abilities, such as the ability to perceive their surroundings. Their abilities also enable them to begin to interact with their parents. Figure 6.1 summarises the developmental changes discussed in this chapter.

Parent–child interactions play a central role in the development of parent–child relationships. Irrespective of the age of the child, the parent–child relationship will usually be such that the parents will:

- Require psychological care in the form of emotional support
- Be able to make a positive contribution to the nursing care of their child

Good communication is crucial to good nursing care of children just as it is crucial to good nursing care in general. Young children sometimes have difficulty expressing themselves verbally and understanding language. Some of these difficulties can be reduced by creating a supportive context and providing non-verbal cues to help children understand what is being said.

Children's ideas about what happens inside their bodies and about the causes of illness are not always the same as those of adults. In order to communicate successfully with children about illness, their existing level of understanding should be established. The nurse can then try to build on this existing knowledge and correct any misconceptions which may be causing distress.

References

Bibace R and Walsh M E (1980) Development of children's concepts of illness. *Pediatrics*, **66**: 912–917

Birns B (1965) Individual differences in human neonates' responses to stimulation. *Child Development*, **36**: 249–256

Bloom L M (1973) *One Word at a Time: The Use of Single Word Utterances Before Syntax*. The Hague: Mouton.

Bower T G R (1979) *Human Development*. San Francisco: Freeman.

Bowlby J (1958) The nature of the child's tie to his mother. *International Journal of Psychoanalysis*, **39**: 350–373.

Bowlby J (1973) *Attachment and Loss, vol. 2: Separation, Anxiety and Anger*. London: Hogarth Press.

Brain D J and Maclay I (1968) Controlled study of mothers and children in hospital. *British Medical Journal*, **i**: 278–280.

Brewster A B (1982) Chronically ill hospitalized children's concepts of their illness. *Pediatrics*, **69**: 355–362.

Carpenter G (1974) Mother's face and the newborn. *New Scientist*, **61** : 742–744.

Consumers' Association (1980) *Children in Hospital*. London: Consumers' Association.

Crawford-Blitzer E Zuckerman B Pozen J T and Blitzer P H (1983) Another myth: reduced hospital visiting by inner-city mothers. *Pediatrics*, **71**: 504–509.

Crider C (1981) Children's conceptions of the body interior. In: *New Directions for Child Development: Children's Conceptions of Health, Illness, and Bodily Functions*, eds. Bibace R and Walsh M. San Francisco: Jossey-Bass.

Donaldson M (1978) *Children's Minds*. London: Fontana.

Donaldson M L (1986) *Children's Explanations: A Psycholinguistic Study*. Cambridge: Cambridge University Press.

Eiser C and Patterson D (1983) 'Slugs and snails and puppy-dog tails' – children's ideas about the inside of their bodies. *Child: Care, Health and Development*, **9**: 233–240.

Friedman S L Jacobs B S and Werthmann M W (1981) Sensory processing in pre- and full-term infants in the neonatal period. In: *Preterm Birth and Psychological Development*, eds. Friedman S L and Sigman M. London: Academic Press.

Kister M C and Patterson C J (1980) Children's conceptions of the causes of illness: understanding of contagion and use of immanent justice. *Child Development*, **51**: 839–846.

Klaus M H, Jerauld R, Kreger N, McAlpine W, Steffa M and Kennell J H (1972) Maternal attachment - importance of the first postpartum days. *New England Journal of Medicine*, **286**: 460–463.

MacFarlane A (1977) *The Psychology of Childbirth*. London: Fontana.

Macnamara J (1977) From sign to language. In: *Language, Learning and Thought*, ed. Macnamara J. New York: Academic Press.

Meltzoff A N and Moore M K (1977) Imitation of facial and manual gestures. *Science*, **198**: 75–80.

Muller D J Harris P J and Wattley L (1986) *Nursing Children: Psychology, Research and Practice*. London: Harper & Row.

Myers B (1982) Early intervention using Brazelton training with middle-class mothers and fathers of newborns. *Child Development*, **53**: 462–471.

Parke R D (1981) *Fathering*. London: Fontana.

Perrin E C and Gerrity P S (1981) There's a demon in your belly: children's understanding of illness. *Pediatrics*, **67**: 841–849.

Porter C (1974) Grade school children's perceptions of their internal body parts. *Nursing Research*, **23**: 384–391.

Poster E C (1983) Stress immunization: techniques to help children cope with hospitilization. *Maternal Child Nursing Journal*, **12**: 119–134.

Richards M P M (1978) Possible effects of early separation on later development of children – rereview. In: *Separation and Special Care Baby Units*, eds. Brimblecombe F S W, Richards M P M and Roberton N R C London: Heinemann.

Robertson J and Robertson J (1968) *Young Children in Brief Separation: John*. London: Tavistock Child Development Research Unit.

Rodin J (1983) *Will This Hurt?* RCN Research Series. London: Royal College of Nursing.

Ross D M and Ross S A (1984) Childhood pain: the school-aged child's viewpoint. *Pain*, **20**: 179–191.

Rutter M (1981) *Maternal Deprivation Reassessed*. Harmondsworth: Penguin.

Schaffer H R and Emerson P E (1964) The development of social attachments in infancy. *Monographs of the Society for Research in Child Development*, Vol. 29, no. 94.

Schaffer R (1977) *Mothering*. London: Fontana.

Slater A, Morison V and Rose D (1983) Perception of shape by the new-born baby. *British Journal of Developmental Psychology*, **1**: 135–142.

Slater A, Rose D and Morison V (1984) New born infants' perception of similarities and differences between two- and three-dimensional stimuli. *British Journal of Developmental Psychology*, **2**: 287–294.

Sluckin W, Herbert M and Sluckin A (1983) *Maternal Bonding*. Oxford: Basil Blackwell.

Stenbak E (1986) *Care of Children in Hospital*. Copenhagen: World Health Organization.

Stern D (1977) *The First Relationship: Infant and Mother*. London: Fontana.

Stern M and Hildebrandt K A (1986) Premature stereotyping: effects on mother-infant interaction. *Child Development*, **57**: 308–315.

Tizard B (1977) *Adoption: A Second Chance*. London: Open Books.

Tizard B and Hughes M (1984) *Young Children Learning: Talking and Thinking at Home and at School*. London: Fontana.

Trevarthen C (1977) Descriptive analyses of infant communicative behaviour. In: *Studies in Mother-Infant Interaction*, ed. Schaffer H R. London: Academic Press.

Wertheimer M (1961) Psychomotor coordination of auditory-visual space at birth. *Science*, **134**: 1692.

Wolff P H (1963) Observations on the development of smiling. In: *Determinants of Infant Behaviour*, ed. Foss B M, vol. 2. London: Methuen.

7
Pain and Pain Management

Pain is both a psychological and a physiological phenomenon, so the experience of pain cannot be understood either from a purely physiological or a purely psychological perspective. Caring for people suffering from pain requires an understanding of both the physiology and psychology of pain and how the two interact.

The purpose of this chapter is to provide information about pain and its management so that a nurse can reduce the suffering of patients in her care.

The chapter is divided into three sections. The first section explains how pain is caused in terms of the underlying physiological and psychological mechanisms. The second section examines the management of patients with acute pain, in particular, those in accident and emergency departments and those undergoing preoperative preparation in advance of surgery. The third section provides an account of the management of patients with chronic pain, with special reference to stress reducing techniques.

THE CAUSES OF PAIN

The ability to feel pain is very important. The few people who are born without the sensation of pain are at a tremendous disadvantage: they burn and hurt themselves without noticing. Pain is a protective message to the brain to alert the person to do something about the cause of the pain. Of course, pain is not always good, and in most nursing contexts it is important to alleviate it. Not only is pain distressing but also the stress which it causes can inhibit recovery. Pain management is an important aspect of nursing, and effective management requires the nurse to understand how pain is produced.

Pain receptors are important to the experience of pain. However, physical damage or stimulation of pain receptors does not necessarily lead to the experience of pain and, similarly, the experience of pain can occur without any physical damage. The reason is that certain events happen between the pain receptor and the sensation of pain and these events alter whether or not a stimulus is sensed as pain. The following account of pain perception starts with the peripheral pain receptors and traces the sequence of events which occurs until pain is perceived in the brain.

The periphery: pain receptors

In the skin and in all parts of the body apart from the brain can be found the free endings of nerves which have small-diameter fibres (A-delta and C fibres) leading from them. These free nerve endings are the pain receptors which when stimulated can give rise to the sensation of pain. The stimulation can occur in various forms: chemical, pressor and electrical.

Drugs which inhibit the stimulation of these free nerve endings are called *peripherally acting analgesics*. The most commonly used peripherally acting analgesics are aspirin and paracetamol. Both aspirin and paracetamol have a *ceiling effect*, i.e. there is a level beyond which an increase in dosage has no increased effect on pain relief, which means that there is a limit to the effectiveness of these analgesics. Aspirin and paracetamol do not relieve very intense pain, although they are effective for mild levels of pain. For aspirin, the ceiling dosage is approximately 1 000 mg given every four hours. An advantage of both aspirin and paracetamol is that the body does not adapt to these substances. This means that the effectiveness of pain relief from these drugs does not decline with repeated use over time.

A summary of the features of the most commonly used analgesics is given on page 121.

The spinal cord: the 'gate'

The 'gate theory' of pain was proposed by Melzack and Wall (1965, 1968) and this theory has made a substantial contribution to our understanding of pain. According to this theory, there is a 'gate' or a series of gates throughout the length of the spinal cord. The pain messages which originate from the periphery travel to the gate in the spinal cord; if the gate is open, the pain messages get through to the brain, if the gate is closed, they do not.

Two types of nerve are relevant to the gate theory of pain. First, there are the small-diameter fibres, the A-delta and C fibres, which originate from the pain receptors (see above). Second, there are large-diameter fibres, or A-beta fibres, which are sensory fibres and include those which are sensitive to touch.

Both the large- and small-diameter fibres stimulate so-called *T cells*. T cells are located in the spinal cord and, when activated, pass the pain message up to the brain. However, the activity of the T cells is affected by another type of cell located in an adjacent part of the spinal cord, the *substantia gelatinosa*. Activity in the substantia gelatinosa inhibits the effect of both the small and large fibres on the T cells and thus, inhibits the transmission of the pain message up to the brain.

The large-diameter fibres also increase the activity of the substantia gelatinosa, whereas the small-diameter fibres decrease it. The arrangement is shown in figure 7.1.

The overall effect, then, is that large-diameter sensory fibres have an inhibitory effect on the T cells. This inhibitory effect is not immediate, as it takes time for the large-diameter cells to arouse the substantia gelatinosa. Thus, the initial effect of the large-diameter cells may be a temporary increase in T cell activity and hence the sensation of pain.

The gate then closes gradually with repeated stimulation of the large fibres. Under normal circumstances, however, the gate does not fully close, and the reason for this is that nerve cells adapt to repeated stimulation, that is they fire less rapidly after continued stimulation. The small-diameter nerves, i.e. the fibres carrying the pain message, adapt very slowly. On the other hand, large-diameter fibres, those carrying the sensory message, adapt quite quickly. The consequence of this is that, under

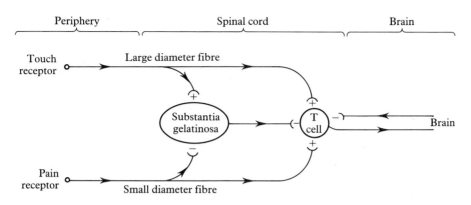

Fig. 7.1 Illustration of the spinal cord mechanisms underlying the gate theory of pain.

Activity in the peripheral nerve either excites ('+') or inhibits ('−') other cells. Once the substantia gelatinosa becomes activated the T cell is inhibited so that pain messages are not transmitted to the brain.

normal circumstances, the large-diameter fibres do not have a long-term inhibitory effect on the sensation of tissue damage because stimulation from touch adapts whereas stimulation from pain does not. However, if the touch receptors and their associated fibres are not allowed to adapt because the stimulation is constantly varied, touch will have a long-term effect of reducing pain by closing the spinal gate.

Transcutaneous electrical nerve stimulation (TENS) is a technique based on the idea that large-diameter nerves can be prevented from adapting by varying the stimulation, and can thus decrease the sensation of pain. In TENS, electrodes are placed on the skin over the painful area and a small, pulsed electrical current is passed between the electrodes. The current has to be pulsed (i.e. in bursts) rather than continuous to prevent the large-diameter nerves from adapting to the stimulation. This variable stimulation of the sensory nerves leads to a gradual activation of the substantia gelatinosa and so inhibits the effects of the small pain fibres on the T cells. In practical terms, the electrical stimulation closes the gate so that pain is no longer perceived. The pain-relieving effect persists for some time after the electrical stimulation has finished.

TENS has been found to be a useful tool in pain management in certain instances, typically where pain is localised (i.e. the pain messages enter at a particular level of the spinal cord so that sensory fibres can be stimulated at that level too). For example, TENS is effective for women in labour with back pain, but not effective for women in labour who have lower abdominal pain, where the pain messages are not localised.

The gate theory of pain is a useful way of explaining some abnormal pain phenomena (Melzack and Wall, 1968). If the large-diameter sensory nerves are selectively destroyed (which can occur in some diabetic and alcohol-related conditions) the substantia gelatinosa is no longer activated and so no longer inhibits the stimulation of T cells. Under such circumstances, the gate is left wide open. The resting level of small-diameter fibre activity which occurs in the absence of nerve-ending stimulation is sufficient to stimulate the T cells. This forms the basis for intense pathological pain which has no actual source, e.g. phantom limb pain following amputation.

In figure 7.1, an arrow is shown going from 'higher control processes' to the gate. Higher control processes, which include mood (e.g. anxiety and depression) and level of attention, can alter the opening or closing of the gate. This higher-level effect on the gate comes about through neural pathways descending from the brain to the spinal cord. The ability of the mind to close the gate has clear survival value. A hunter running away from a lion who tears his leg on some sharp thorns will not have time to stop and attend to his wounds. Just as pain perception is useful to human survival, so sometimes is the ability to ignore pain.

The brain: higher level control of pain

Higher-level processes can affect pain perception in two ways: they can affect the gate and they can affect the perception of pain within the brain itself. The T cells in the spinal cord transmit impulses to the brain where they may or may not be interpreted as the sensation of pain. There are a number of factors which determine the intensity of pain experience at this level.

Attention and distraction

If one is preoccupied, one is less likely to feel pain. Footballers often do not feel the pain caused by a kick during a football match, but if an equivalent kick was given in the street they would certainly feel pain. People escaping from a burning plane are often unaware of injuries to their legs despite those injuries being quite severe. Distraction is a useful nursing technique which can be used to control pain, both chronic and acute.

Perceived control

Removing a splinter seems to hurt a lot less if one gets it out oneself; it seems to hurt much more if someone else is digging around with a needle. The reason for this is that the perceived control over the pain seems to reduce the pain experience. In general, the more that people feel that they are able to control what is going on, the less pain they feel. Other psychological benefits of perceived control or self-determination were described in chapter 1.

In one sense, perceived control appears to be the opposite of distraction. For example, when taking a splinter out oneself, one is focusing on the splinter rather than being distracted from it. In another sense, taking out the splinter is a kind of distraction in that the focus is on the problem of getting the splinter out rather than the pain.

Perceived control is related to the problem-solving approach of coping with pain. Some people have a coping style where they try to do as much as possible to learn about the pain and deal with it themselves. Other people prefer a more passive role where the main aim is distraction (Martelli et al, 1987). Thus, both distraction (trying to pretend the pain is not happening) and perceived control (focusing on the pain and controlling it) can lead to pain reduction.

Expectancy and hypnosis

Research (reviewed in Kirsch, in press) shows that when people expect to feel pain, they are more likely to experience it, but when they expect not to feel pain, they are more likely not to. This *expectancy* is a strong mechanism thought to be responsible for placebo effects in pain relief. Expectancy effects also add to any analgesic effect of a drug.

Placebo pain relief occurs when the patient is given a physiologically inactive substance and then reports that his pain has reduced. If a patient receives relief from a placebo, it does not mean that the pain was in some sense unreal. It simply means that the expectancy which was generated by the placebo treatment is counteracting the pain.

Research (reviewed by Kirsch, in press) shows that placebo 'morphine' is more effective than placebo 'aspirin'. Because aspirin and paracetamol are available without prescription they are often undervalued by patients who ask for something stronger. In fact, aspirin may well be the most effective drug for a patient's condition. Telling the patient that the drug is aspirin may reduce the expectancy effects of pain relief, and therefore it is sometimes better to give aspirin and simply call it a 'good pain killer'.

Hypnosis and post-hypnotic control of pain involve suggesting to the patient, while he is under hypnosis, that he does not feel pain. Good hypnotic subjects (about one third of the population) obtain pain relief from hypnosis; poor hypnotic subjects (the remaining two-thirds of the population) do not. It is thought that the expectancy effect is the mechanism underlying hypnosis.

The effectiveness of pain reduction through any of these expectancy-based techniques (hypnosis or placebo treatment) varies between patients. It is possible to carry out painful procedures (such as surgery) under hypnosis and to obtain powerful pain relief with placebos, but these techniques are not always effective.

It is incorrect to suppose that placebo pain relief is most effective for 'neurotic' patients or those who have some psychological problem. On the contrary, research (Kirsch, in press) shows that there is only a weak correlation between personality-type and placebo pain relief. Furthermore, the degree to which placebos have been effective in the past for a particular person does not accurately predict whether placebos will act for him in the future. In summary, the research shows that it is difficult to predict who will react well to placebo pain relief.

Anxiety

Evidence shows that people who are anxious report more pain than people who are not anxious (Weisenberg, 1980). Anxiety may increase pain by focusing attention on the pain and providing a negative interpretation of the pain-causing event. Anxiety may also intensify pain by increasing central nervous system (CNS) activity. Drugs which reduce anxiety by depressing CNS activity (e.g. barbiturates and alcohol) also have the effect of reducing pain. These are called *adjuvant analgesics*.

Techniques for reducing anxiety were discussed in chapters 2 and 3. For example, a nurse can reduce a patient's anxiety by providing the information the patient wants about his condition, so effective communication with patients is important to reduce the experience of pain.

Interpretation of cause of pain

There is evidence that the interpretation placed on physical damage affects the experience of pain. Soldiers who are wounded in battle can have a positive attitude towards their wounds because they remove them from the danger of death. Beecher (1956) found that wounded soldiers asked for much less pain relief than civilian patients with equivalent physical damage caused by operations. People who have strong negative attitudes to being in hospital are more likely to feel pain.

Depression

Feelings of depression and the experience of pain tend to go together, though the mere correlation of depression and pain does not make it clear which is causing which. Romano and Turner (1985), however, conclude that there is research evidence supporting the following four claims.

1. Depression increases the perception of pain
2. Pain is a stressor which causes depression
3. Some people experience pain and depression as being, in some sense, equivalent
4. Pain and depression share similar biochemical processes (for more detail see Beutler et al, 1986).

In other words, there is a two-way causal relationship between pain and depression, each influencing the other.

Antidepressant drugs can reduce the experience of pain. Like sedative and anxiolytic drugs, antidepressants are classified as adjuvant analgesics when used to control pain. Furthermore, nursing actions which discourage the development of depression (e.g. actions which prevent the development of learned helplessness, see chapter 1) are likely to reduce pain.

Drug effects

Endorphins (endogenously-produced opioid substances) are opiate substances produced by the body which occur naturally in the brain and which reduce the sensation of pain. Endorphins are one of the body's own mechanisms for reducing pain. It is thought that expectancy or placebo effects operate at least partially through the production of endorphins.

Some recent research by Bandura et al (1987) throws light on the physiological mechanisms underlying psychological techniques of pain control, using the drug naloxone which prevents the formation of endorphins. Bandura et al gave one group of people psychological training in pain control, and another group no training. Half the people in the psychologically-trained group were then given naxolone. The naloxone reduced the pain-relieving effects of psychological training, but it did not abolish them to the level of the untrained group. Thus, it would appear that psychological mechanisms of pain control operate partially but not entirely through the production of endorphins.

The *narcotic analgesics* are chemically similar to endorphins and also have a pain-relieving effect. These narcotic analgesics mimic the effect of the naturally-occurring endorphins. The best known narcotic analgesics are codeine and morphine, the latter being the more powerful, but there are many others all of which have a similar effect on pain perception.

The site of action of a centrally-acting drug like morphine should be contrasted with the site of action of a peripherally-acting analgesic like aspirin. Also, the biochemical properties of the peripheral and narcotic analgesics are quite different. Unlike peripheral analgesics, people adapt to narcotic analgesics so that over a period of time a greater dosage is needed to have the same pain-relieving effect. Also, there is a risk of drug dependency and drug abuse with narcotic analgesics, whereas this risk does not occur with the peripherally-acting analgesics.

Earlier, it was suggested that placebo pain reduction adds to the active effect of an analgesic drug. Some authors believe that narcotic drugs have an effect largely due to expectancy and distraction. Beecher (1957, p.152) wrote, 'Narcotics really alter pain perception very little but do produce a bemused state, comparable to distraction'. Narcotics do not actually remove the sensation of pain, but they make the pain sensation 'less bothersome'. Recent evidence in support of the view that narcotic pain relief acts primarily through psychological reappraisal of the pain is reviewed by Kirsch (in press). For example, the gaseous anaesthetic nitrous oxide will increase pain if the subject expects nitrous oxide to make him more sensitive to stimulation but will decrease pain if he expects nitrous oxide to be an analgesic. Kirsch concludes that 'The pain-relieving effects of some active drugs may be entirely due to expectancy'. These findings suggest that at least part of the effectiveness of a narcotic analgesic is due to psychological mechanisms. This does not mean that pain relief is any less real: it simply points to the importance of psychological factors in the experience and management of pain.

The three classes of pain-relieving drug, are summarised below.

1. *Peripherally-acting analgesics* or non-narcotic analgesics, (such as aspirin and paracetamol) operate on the free nerve endings. Both aspirin and paracetamol have a ceiling on their effectiveness which for both drugs is at a dose of about 1000 mg every four hours. The body does not adapt to their use. Apart from inhibiting the activity of free nerve endings, aspirin has positive and negative side-effects. It is anti-inflammatory and antipyretic (i.e. it lowers body temperature). Aspirin sometimes has negative side-effects, most commonly causing gastric problems such as gastritis and ulcers. Due to the negative side-effects not everyone can tolerate aspirin, and the common alternative is paracetamol. Paracetamol is antipyretic but not anti-inflammatory. It does not have the side-effect of causing gastric irritation and bleeding. However, overdosing with paracetamol is very dangerous; high levels of paracetamol, particularly when taken in combination with alchohol, can cause liver and kidney damage.

2. *Narcotic analgesics*, or centrally-acting analgesics, operate within the brain and mimic the effect of endorphins. At high dosages these drugs cause loss of consciousness. Moderately high dosages can produce greater analgesia than occurs with the peripherally-acting analgesics. However, adaptation occurs so over time an increasingly high dose is needed to maintain analgesia. These drugs are potentially addictive, and are not available without prescription. The narcotic analgesics differ among themselves in terms of their potency (e.g. morphine is stronger than codeine), their duration of action (e.g. pethidine is shorter-acting than morphine) and the particular type of endorphin receptor they stimulate in the brain.

3. *Adjuvant analgesics* reduce pain either through their effect on body functions which give rise to pain sensation (e.g. antispasmodic medications, which cause muscle relaxation) or through their effect on higher processes (e.g. sedative hypnotics, anxiolytic medications and antidepressants).

All analgesic drugs, peripheral, narcotic and adjuvant, can reduce pain through expectancy mechanisms independently of any analgesic effect of the drug.

PAIN MANAGEMENT

From a nursing perspective, pain management can be dealt with under two headings.

1. Management of acute pain
2. Management of chronic pain

However, before discussing the management of acute and chronic pain, there is one important general point which should be remembered when dealing with any patient in pain. In order to manage pain, it is first necessary to assess pain. When assessing a patient's experience of pain, it is essential to believe the patient.

Pain experience does not have a simple one-to-one relationship with the stimulation of pain receptors. Because of this, people who have the same degree of physical damage can experience different levels of pain. These individual differences in pain perception are of two kinds. First, some people have a lower *threshold* of pain than others, i.e. what is painful to some people may not be painful to others. Second, some people have a lower *tolerance* of pain than others, i.e. they are more sensitive to pain and can tolerate it less well than others.

When all is said and done, pain is something the patient experiences. The nurse does not experience the patient's pain, and it is not her job to decide for the patient how much pain he is suffering. The nurse's assessment of a patient's pain should start from the assumption that the patient is telling the truth. The following two examples illustrate why it is so important to believe the patient.

- John was a 21-year-old undergraduate who broke his leg while playing football. After the leg had been set in plaster, he was told to try putting pressure on the broken leg. John was told that it might hurt a bit but he found the pain intense. He told this to the nurses who implied that he was just making a fuss. Eventually, it was found that John's leg had been set incorrectly and needed resetting.

- Sally Hopkins was a mother of three children expecting her fourth baby. She began experiencing severe abdominal pain and was admitted to hospital. It was assumed that the pain had something to do with her pregnancy, but there was no evidence of any physical problem. Mrs Hopkins repeatedly asked for pain relief. She was told by the ward sister to 'Stop making a fuss; what do you think labour is going to be like if you make such a fuss about a little thing like this'. The pain was intense and Mrs Hopkins was so distressed that she was unable to say, 'I have had three babies and this pain is much worse than labour'. Mrs Hopkins was extremely upset by the way she was treated by the nursing staff. Eventually, the consultant agreed to an exploratory operation. He found a perforated gut which necessitated the removal of 12 inches of colon. Mrs Hopkins was angry and bitter about the way she was treated by the nursing staff and says that she will never forget the experience, and will always remember the ward sister with a feeling of loathing.

The importance of accepting at face value a patient's report of pain cannot be stressed enough. Some people may make more of a fuss than others but, then, they may experience more pain. There is a legal principle that it is better to let off a guilty person than wrongly imprison an innocent one. In the same way, in nursing it is better to believe someone who is not telling the truth than disbelieve someone who is telling the truth. Biases in person perception (see chapter 4) must not be allowed to bias the assessment of a patient's reported pain. The nurse should avoid statements which indicate that she thinks that the patient is making a fuss. She should also avoid statements which the patient might interpret as her thinking that he is making a fuss. For example, the statements 'You seem rather sensitive to pain' or 'You seem to have quite a low pain threshold' can easily be misinterpreted as 'You are making too much of a fuss about it'.

As stated before, anxiety increases pain. However, it is quite unfair to a patient to say that he is anxious and therefore that his pain can be ignored. Patients who are labelled 'anxious' by nursing staff may suffer needlessly. Not only are their symptoms ignored leading to an incorrect diagnosis, but they are also given insufficient care for their pain.

How good are nurses at finding out about a patient's pain experience? A research study by Camp and O'Sullivan (1987) showed that nurses documented less than 50 per cent of what the patient reported about pain. This figure indicates that some nurses are either not giving sufficient credence to or not attaching sufficient importance to the patient's reports of pain.

Finally, it is important to stress that pain is a protective message which gives information that something is wrong. Pain is not just something to be controlled: it also gives information which may be useful in diagnosis so the nurse should help the doctor to arrive at accurate understanding of the patient's pain for purpose of diagnosis.

Assessing pain

Level of pain

A first step in assessing pain is to find out exactly how painful the pain is. An easy way to do this is to use a 'painometer'. A painometer is simply a scale written on a card which the patient uses to indicate his level of pain, for example:

I have no pain ——————————— My pain is as bad as I can imagine
                 1 2 3 4 5 6 7 8 9 10

The patient is asked to indicate where his pain falls on the scale.

Alternative types of painometer allow the patient to indicate the level of his pain in terms of named categories, e.g.:

0 = No pain
1 = Mild
2 = Discomforting

3 = Distressing
4 = Horrible
5 = Excruciating

(From the McGill Pain Questionnaire [Melzack, 1975])

Obviously, the painometer is not a very accurate assessment tool. People who have experienced very intense pain (such as childbirth) may give a lower estimate for the same sensation than people who have not experienced such intense pain. Nevertheless, the painometer is sufficiently accurate to be a useful indicator.

Temporal pattern of pain

For the purpose of diagnosis, it is often useful to ascertain changes in pattern of pain over a period of time. It is also helpful to determine temporal changes for the purpose of pain management, particularly for chronic pain (see below).

Type of pain

Pain varies in its character, and people use words to characterise the different types of pain. Typical examples of words used to describe pain are 'tingling', 'aching', 'gnawing', 'stabbing', 'burning' and 'shooting'. Different types of pain are sometimes associated with different physical conditons, so knowing the type of pain can help in diagnosis. The McGill Pain Questionnaire (Melzack, 1975) was devised to provide a detailed assessment of type of pain, and has been found to be quite useful in distinguishing different types of underlying pathology (Taylor, 1986).

Talking to the patient when assessing pain

After assessing the level of pain the nurse should try to find out about the temporal pattern and type of pain. Even if these questions are not asked in order to carry out any specific nursing action, it is nevertheless important to find out about the patient's experience of pain. The information may be used at a later date and, in any case, asking these questions helps build up a therapeutic relationship between patient and nurse so that the patient feels that his pain is understood and accepted for what it is. Patients can have difficulty in identifying the location, type and temporal pattern of pain (Camp and O'Sullivan, 1987) so skilled questionning may be needed.

A useful response to a patient's report of pain is an exploratory-reflecting statement (see chapter 2). The nurse should reply with something like, 'Is it hurting more than before?' or 'What does the pain feel like?' Such exploratory-reflecting statements show that she accepts the patient's report of pain but would like to find out more about it. The conversation should, of course, be conducted with the appropriate use of eye contact and other active listening cues (see chapter 2).

It is particularly important for the nurse to question children about their feelings of pain and to make it absolutely clear that she understands that they are in pain. Children may cry and scream, believing it to be the only way of indicating that pain is being experienced (Brewster, 1982). Questioning about pain in an exploratory-reflecting way is a useful way of getting the message across that screaming is not needed.

ACUTE PAIN

Acute pain is pain where a gradual reduction in intensity is expected over a period of time. The two most common situations for nursing patients with acute pain are in accident and emergency departments and on surgical wards. The major difference between these locations is that in accident and emergency the patient is in pain without the nurse having had the opportunity of preparing him for this pain, whereas on a surgical ward, there is the opportunity for nurses to prepare the patient.

'Accident and emergency': acute pain without the opportunity for preparation

Patients who are admitted to hospital in pain are usually frightened about what has happened to them and anxious about what is going to happen. Hospitals are stressful places and feelings of anxiety will only exacerbate the experience of pain, so the first thing the nurse should do is to provide reassurance.

Statements like, 'We are here to look after you', 'Is there anything you want?' or 'Now we are going to try to make you more comfortable' are useful reassuring words which do not mean much in themselves but indicate to the patient that he is in contact with caring people. In addition to talking to the patient, the nurse can also use expressive physical contact (e.g. simply touching the patient). A good therapeutic relationship may well reduce pain experience for the patient, a point which is returned to later in this chapter. Last, and by no means least, the simple fact that a nurse is present with the patient and attending to him will often reduce his anxiety and discomfort.

The nurse should not draw attention to the experience of pain; recall that distraction from and expectancy about pain both affect the pain experience. It is best not to say, 'You look as though you have been in the wars' or 'You have got yourself into a bit of a mess haven't you?' Humorous statements about the patient's condition are generally not recommended.

Some patients naturally attempt to distract themselves. Others can be helped by employing the technique of *guided imagery*. In guided imagery, the nurse encourages the patient to think about something pleasing while a painful procedure is being carried out. Squeezing someone's hand falls into this category of distraction, though any form of distractor will do.

Beales (1979) carried out a study of the effects of distraction on children attending a hospital accident and emergency department. Twelve children (aged from five to 13 years) were observed during suturing of a wound. The nurses successfully hid the first suture from the child's sight and engaged the child's attention through conversation. Unfortunately, the casualty doctor often said something like, 'There, that didn't hurt, did it'. In all cases, the child expressed pain on subsequent sutures. Beales found in other cases that children experienced more pain if medical staff or parents commented on the 'unpleasantness' of the wound, for example, by saying, 'Oh dear, you have got a mess there, haven't you'. Beales argues that although medical staff justify giving children information about pain by not wanting to deceive them, this practice may enhance the experience of pain. Furthermore, non-verbal communication from parents that the procedure is painful may also enhance the experience of pain. Finally,

Beales reported that children often showed distress when their case was being discussed between their parents and the medical staff, and this may have been due to children misunderstanding and exaggerating the adults' conversation.

There are two points to note about Beales' study. The first is that it was carried out on children. Children are more hypnotically susceptible than adults, and so we would expect that expectations of pain or lack of pain would be more strongly self-fulfilling than with adults. The second point is that the pain caused by suturing is quite low when compared with some other procedures. Distraction tends to be useful only where pain sensation is relatively low (McCaul and Malott, 1984). Where pain is more intense, other techniques for pain management such as perceived control over the pain may also be useful.

In the perceived control or problem-solving approach to pain management, the person in pain tries to regain control over the situation and the pain by finding out what the cause is and doing something about it. People who have a high need for information prefer to be given information about the techniques involved in medical procedures. Such information would also help allay their anxiety about unknown future events, thereby reducing their pain. The information also acts as a kind of distraction in that the patient can focus on what is being done rather than the pain itself.

There are two ways in which a nurse can help a patient manage pain through perceived control in an accident and emergency department. The first is simply by providing information about what is going to happen and the reasons for the various actions or treatments to be undergone. A second way is to involve the patient in his care. Particularly with older children, the nurse can ask the patient to hold the end of a bandage or sticking plaster or to hold a limb in a particular position. The nurse can thank the patient and say something like, 'You have really done that well', to give the impression that he is acting competently in the situation.

The extent to which the patient should be distracted through injury-irrelevant or injury-relevant conversation or action depends on the patient. To make the correct decision, the nurse needs to ascertain the patient's need for information on the one hand, and his need to be helpless in a traumatic situation on the other. This decision can only by made if the patient is able to communicate with the nurse and the nurse pays attention to the kind of psychological needs which he is currently expressing. If the patient has a high need for control, he is more likely to seek injury-relevant conversation.

One advantage of giving injury-relevant information is that patients may have incorrect assumptions about what is going to happen. Injury-relevant information helps reduce undue anxiety caused by incorrectly held beliefs about treatment.

Patients who are in very severe pain will find that their ability to communicate is hampered. Under such circumstances, closed rather than open questions should be asked. 'Small talk' should not be made to be an additional burden for the patient. In particular, the nurse should pay attention to whether the patient is breathless, as talking is particularly distressing to someone who is dyspnoeic.

Patients who are in great acute pain are often prescribed analgesics. Narcotic analgesics can be used under such circumstances because they are very powerful and because there is little likelihood of dependency setting in if they are taken only for a matter of days rather than weeks. The disadvantage of narcotic analgesics is that some time is necessary for the drug to pass the blood-brain barrier to their site of action (up to 30 minutes) so that the effects are not instantaneous. However, there is often an instantaneous pain relief which may be due to a placebo effect. The instantaneous effect which addicts experience on injection of heroin cannot be explained pharmacologically.

As stated above, research (reviewed in Kirsch, in press) shows that 'morphine' placebos have a greater effect than 'aspirin' placebos. Clearly, the patient's confidence in the pain-relieving technique will alter his perception of pain, so the nurse should provide analgesics with statements like, 'It is very good for pain', which will help the patient to feel confident in the medication.

One of the problems of managing an accident and emergency department is that patients do not arrive by appointment, so inevitably there are times when patients have to wait. The experience of waiting can provoke anxiety in a patient because he does not know how long he is going to wait or, indeed, whether he has simply been forgotten. If nurses discuss with the patient how long he is likely to have to wait and explain, if appropriate, that there are other patients who are critically ill and need treatment, many patients find the waiting easier. Another technique to reduce anxiety is to move patients from one room to another to give the impression of progression through the department. However, the general principle is that explanation of how the accident and emergency department operates can relieve anxiety at what is generally a very traumatic time for patients.

Children in casualty

Children are particularly prone to misunderstanding the purpose of treatments. Brewster (1982) found that many five- and six-year-olds thought that nurses and doctors carried out medical procedures to punish them, though by the age of seven these children appreciated that treatment was designed to help recovery. Beales et al (1983) report that, up until the age of 11 years, children have difficulty in understanding that treatments which are unpleasant in the short term can have long-term benefits. So the nurse should explain to children what is being done, assuming that there is time, even for the most obvious treatments. Also, the nurse should say to younger children something like, 'You are a very good boy, aren't you, Johnny?' to show that there is no punishment involved. It is worth noting that the community nurse and school nurse can both play an educational role in preparing children for the possibility of treatment in a casualty department.

If distraction is not being used or is not working, it is important to communicate to the child awareness of his pain or discomfort, for example by saying, 'I know it isn't very nice but it will be better in a minute'. Brewster (1982) found that many children younger than 10 years old thought that the nurses would not know they were in pain unless they cried or screamed.

Children usually arrive in the casualty department with their parents. Research (Ross and Ross, 1984) shows that children find their parents' presence a great help when they are in pain, and thus they should not be separated from them. It is important to reassure parents about their child's condition and treatment as parental anxiety can be communicated non-verbally to children. Such reassurance should involve giving the parents information, listening to their anxieties and providing answers to their queries. It is entirely wrong and very patronising to assume that parents will 'get upset', and so prevent them from being present while their children are being treated.

Surgery: acute pain with the opportunity for preparation

Patients are admitted to hospital with a variety of attitudes towards their operation. To a businessman or self-employed worker, surgery may mean loss of earnings or loss of career potential. To a busy mother, surgery can mean anxiety about arrangements for her children. However, for people who are lonely, surgery has positive aspects and may be less daunting; it may mean companionship and being looked after by caring nurses.

As the attitude towards a painful event affects pain experience, a nurse should initially assess the effect of surgery on the patient's normal, non-hospitalised life. In particular, the nurse should be sensitive to his 'non-hospital' needs while in hospital, such as the need for contact with colleagues or relatives, and for information about children.

Because patients are admitted before the surgery takes place, there is usually the opportunity for preoperative preparation. There are several research studies which show that pschological preparation for surgery can have a beneficial effect on post-operative pain experience and recovery. The exact form of psychological preparation (i.e. what and how the patient is told) differs between the studies, and this leads to difficulty in evaluating this body of research, specifically in being certain what form of preparation is most beneficial.

One of the earliest studies was carried out by Egbert, Battit, Welch and Bartlett (1964) who prepared patients for surgery by means of a careful and continuing process of rapport-building, with information given by the patient's own anaesthetist. Such individually-prepared patients required less analgesia and were sent home sooner than unprepared patients. The difficulty in interpreting these results is knowing exactly what was causing the beneficial effect. Was it the rapport, the information or both? Or did the talking by the anaesthetist relax the patient?

Since that early study, there have been a number of others which have examined the effectiveness of preoperative preparation on postoperative recovery and pain experience. Again, a problem in interpreting these studies is that more than one form of preoperative preparation is given at one time. Nevertheless, a likely interpretation is that a number of different types of preoperative preparation work in reducing pain. These fall into three categories: conveying information, providing coping devices and giving relaxation training.

Conveying information

The basic idea behind information-giving is that its long-term, postoperative aim is to reduce stress as stress is harmful to physical recovery. The use of information to reduce stress is sometimes referred to as *stress inoculation*. Langer, Janis and Wolfer (1975) describe it in this way:

- 'According to this conception, such preparatory communications are effective when they arouse a moderate level of anticipatory fear, which leads to constructive 'work of worrying,' i.e. mentally rehearsing the impending threats and developing realistic, self-delivered reassurances that prevent subsequent emotional shocks.' (1975, p. 157)

Preoperative information given by Boore (1978) included discussion on the following.

1. Preoperative preparation on the ward

2. Preoperative starvation and medication

3. The anaesthetic, the induction of anaesthesia, and the recovery room

4. Postoperative circumstances and experience

Both studies (Boore, 1978; Langer et al, 1975) indicate that information can reduce postoperative pain and request for analgesia. In particular, Boore found a reduction of one of the corticosteroid stress hormones in such conditions. Corticosteroids inhibit healing and so lower levels of secretion imply a faster recovery from surgery.

Information in booklet as opposed to interview format has also been found to be effective, leading to enhanced communication with others, fewer incorrect preconceptions, fewer worries and faster recovery (Wallace, 1986).

Just as giving information about postoperative discomfort may lead to lower levels of stress, it is equally true that lack of information is stressful; indeed lack of information is a major complaint about hospitalisation (see chapter 3). If the patient is told that he is going to wear a white gown, have a bath, and wake up feeling sick at a particular time, he has the feeling of control when these events happen and at least knows what is going on.

Coping devices

The basic idea behind a coping device is that the patient either engages in some action to help recovery or shifts his attention to distract himself from the pain. Both techniques give the patient a feeling of control over what is happening. Actions or exercises can help postoperative recovery. Boore (1978) trained patients preoperatively to engage in various postoperative exercises which included:

- How to inspire and expire fully
- How to cough to minimise pain
- Foot, ankle and leg exercises

Other researchers have used distraction or other attention-modifying techniques in preoperative preparation. For example, Wells, Howard, Nowlin and Vargas (1986) provided subjects with skills training which included the following.

- Distraction with pleasant images
- Substitution of negative self-statements with positive self-statements
- Information about pain theory and how pain perception can be controlled

These, and several other studies (e.g. Langer et al, 1975), have shown that coping devices can help reduce reported pain, with the consequence of decreased demand for analgesics.

One point emphasised in chapter 3 is that, when patients are given self-help instructions, the nurse should give reasons for the actions suggested. Patients should not simply be instructed to engage in exercises (as indicated by Boore, 1978) but should be given reasons for those exercises. These are as follows.

1. Patients should practise breathing using the diaphragm (a hand placed on the stomach should rise up and down when breathing if this is being done correctly) and the lower part of the rib cage. Such deep breathing helps in the short term to evacuate anaesthetic gases and, in the long term, to reduce the risk of secondary complications such as lung collapse and pneumonia.

2. The anaesthetic causes an increase in mucus production in the bronchial tree and coughing helps expel this. However, coughing is painful particularly after an abdominal operation so patients should be encouraged to cough while holding a pillow pressed against the wound as a support.

3. Foot, ankle and leg exercises reduce the risk of blood clots (thromboses) forming in the deep veins of the leg. Patients should be encouraged to engage in such exercises, particularly if they will be unable to get up for a while.

Relaxation

Preoperative relaxation training is a special sort of coping device. In particular, relaxation can reduce pain caused by muscle contraction and can lower corticosteroid stress hormone levels. Relaxation training can be specific to a group of muscles (for example Boore, 1978, focused on relaxing the abdominal muscles) or it can be general.

Several research studies (Kaplan, Metzger and Jablecki, 1983; Flaherty and Fitzpatrick, 1978) show that preoperative training in general relaxation reduces postoperative pain, though this result is not obtained in all studies (see for example, Mogan, Wells and Robertson, 1985).

Relaxation training is based on several suggestions which are made to the patient, which he then practises and uses, when needed, at a later date. First the patient should be instructed to think about being in a situation which is relaxing or pleasant (this also acts as a distractor to pain). Next he should be asked to breathe deeply and slowly. He is then requested to focus on different parts of the body with the feeling of 'letting go', and letting the muscles relax. He may for example start with his neck and relax different parts of his body, working down to his feet. It is also useful to 'stretch and let go' as a way of encouraging relaxation. Contracting before letting go, e.g. making a ball of the fist, is less effective than stretching. If, in addition to preoperative training, relaxation is to be induced on a particular occasion the nurse should give direct instructions such as, 'You are beginning to feel relaxed now; you feel as though your body is sinking into the bed; your limbs feel very heavy'.

Finally, it must be stressed that although such preparation should occur before surgery, counselling and advice on exercise, distraction, and relaxation should be continued after the operation.

Individual differences

An important weakness of the above studies, and a likely explanation for inconsistent findings in the relaxation studies, is that no account is taken of the patient's personality. These studies are based on the assumption that the same sort of preparatory information will do for everyone. There have been a few studies which have started from the assumption that preoperative preparation needs individualised communication. Auerbach, Kendal, Cuttler and Levitt (1976) investigated pain experience for dental surgery following two types of preparatory information. One type of information, labelled 'external', consisted of telling patients about the general situation in which they were placed (e.g. information about the size and organisation of the dental hospital). The other type of information, 'internal', consisted of giving the patient specific information about what was going to happen to him (e.g. details about how his tooth would be removed). Auerbach et al found that people who typically used internal attributions (i.e. explained events in terms of their own characteristics) experienced less pain if given 'internal' information, whereas those who tended to make external attributions (i.e. explained events in terms of the situation) experienced less pain if given 'external' information.

More recently, Martelli, Auerbach, Alexander and Mercuri (1987) classified patients for oral surgery in terms of which of two ways they had previously used to cope with pain. The first way was to focus on emotional feelings and use techniques of distraction and relaxation to pretend that the pain was not happening. The second way was to concentrate on information about the situation so that the patient felt more in control of the pain which was occurring. Martelli *et al* gave preoperative counselling which, for one group of patients, centred on the first way of coping and for another group, the second way. The results showed that the patients experienced less pain if the type of instruction given was consistent with their preferred style of dealing with pain.

Although there is a scarcity of research on individualising preoperative preparation, a general tenet does seem to be emerging, which is that patients have different ways of coping with pain and that instructions which are consistent with the patient's own way of managing pain produce the best results. Thus, in order to individualise preoperative preparation, the nurse should talk to the patient to assess his normal pattern of coping with pain and his normal pattern for explaining the cause of events. The nurse should then suggest a strategy consistent with patient's normal way of thinking.

There are several reasons why it may be good to match preoperative preparation with the patient's own characteristics. One possibility is that, if the nurse suggests actions which the patient would like to do anyway, the perceived similarity between the nurse and patient leads to the formation of a better therapeutic relationship. And it may be that a good therapeutic relationship helps reduce the experience of pain.

However, it does seem that certain types of patient are better or less able to cope with surgery. Attitude towards surgery has been referred to above but there is also research (reviewed in Wilson-Barnett and Fordham, 1982), which suggests that personality factors are associated with recovery. For example, patients with a negative self-image who are prone to feelings of depression recover less well than those with a positive self-image coupled with the idea that they are 'strong' personalities. The nurse should therefore take special care to avoid inducing feelings of helplessness in those patients who are most at risk of poor self-image and depression (i.e. patients who blame themselves rather than others for their failures.

Wilson-Barnett and Fordham (1982) provide a list of beneficial and harmful factors that effect recovery. These can be summarised as follows.

● Factors aiding recovery	Factors delaying recovery
Youth	Old age
Physical fitness	Other complicating diseases
Good knowledge of illness	Unwillingness to know about illness
Active participation in treatment	Lack of belief in treatment
Good relationship with staff and positive view of rehabilitation by staff	Lack of relevant information from staff
Flexible coping methods	Highly emotional predisposition, passive dependence and persistent denial
Good supportive relationships	Poor family relationships
Good history of employment	Unskilled, irregular employment
Financial security	Financial insecurity and other life stresses

Of course, many of the risk factors in the Wilson-Barnett and Fordham list cannot be changed through nursing action. However, they do illustrate that happy, well-adjusted patients recover best. The reason for this is discussed in chapter 9, as are the implications for health education in the community.

Preoperative preparation of children

Research shows that preoperative preparation of children, as of adults, reduces the stressfulness of hospitilisation (see reviews in Ferguson, 1979; Rodin, 1983; Eiser, 1985). Parents should also be prepared for their child's surgery, since such preparation reduces the parents' feelings of distress and can have the knock-on effect of reducing the child's stress (Skipper and Leonard, 1968; Wolfer and Visintainer, 1979). Furthermore, involvement of parents equips them to play an extremely useful role in preparing their children for surgery (Muller, Harris and Wattley, 1986) and, as chapter 6 emphasised, it is important for parents to participate in the care of their child.

Children (and their parents) should be provided with information about the purpose of treatment and the routine of the ward. As noted above, children's understanding of the purpose of treatment can often be wrong: in particular, nurses should ensure that younger children do not think that their treatment is a punishment. A warm, caring relationship with a nurse can go a long way towards providing a child with reassurance. However, this therapeutic relationship will only develop if the nurse takes time to be with a child, talk to him or even to read him stories, all of which are not always easy on a busy ward.

It is useful for children and their parents to visit the ward a few days before admission to begin to establish relationships with hospital staff. Furthermore, the ward will be a much less frightening place if the child has had the opportunity to visit and play with some of the toys. Children vary considerably in how much in advance they would like to know about a painful procedure (Ross and Ross, 1984), the time ranging from several weeks beforehand to just in advance. However, there is some evidence (Melamed et al, 1976) that the older the child the more effective is long-term preparation. Parents should be encouraged to advise about how their child copes best with anticipated unpleasant events.

Children also can prepare for surgery by playing with toy versions of medical equipment, by dressing up and by playing 'hospitals' with dolls (Rodin, 1983), as play can help children cope with their anxieties about admission (Cassell and Paul, 1967). Schwartz, Albino and Tedesco (1983) show that preoperative play is effective in reducing stress in three- and four-year-olds undergoing dental operations compared with children who did not have the opportunity for play. Sometimes children's play will reveal their concerns about hospital and their understanding of illness, and so it is useful to be watchful so as to provide support or clarification. Parents are better than nurses at interpreting their children's play, so they too should be encouraged to watch such activities.

Children can also be prepared for surgery using story-books or video films (Melamed and Siegel, 1975). The community nurse or health visitor can play an important role in advising parents and providing preparation materials before admission to hospital.

Points to remember in preoperative preparation

Listed below are points to guide the nurse in preparation of patients for surgery.

1. Prior to admission, patients should be provided with written information about hospital procedures and routines.

2. The nurse should try to find time to develop a therapeutic relationship with the patient, and try to find out how the patient typically copes with pain, while also assessing his psychological needs.

3. Information about the operation should be communicated, the patient's ideas on what is going to happen aired, and any misunderstandings corrected. This is particularly important with children.

4. Postoperative pain and postoperative experiences should be discussed before the operation.

5. Coping strategies such as distraction, relaxation or perceived control should be suggested.

6. The patient may find it reassuring if a nurse he knows accompanies him on the journey from the ward to the operating theatre and, if suitable, holds his hand. In the case of children, the parent or parents should be encouraged to accompany the child and the nurse to the operating theatre.

After surgery, a painometer or some more informal technique can be used to assess the patient's pain. Regular analgesia and advice on psychological techniques for pain control should also be provided as appropriate.

MANAGEMENT OF CHRONIC PAIN

The main difference between acute and chronic pain concerns time-scale. In the case of acute pain, there is a characteristic reduction in pain over a period of time. In the case of chronic pain, on the other hand, the experience of pain persists, often with ups and downs, but there is no expectation that the pain will actually go away, at least not by itself.

In the case of acute pain, the message is: 'Hey, take care; let me get better before you do anything rough to me'. But in the case of chronic pain, the message sometimes does not make sense.

Chronic pain is of two sorts. The first is where there is a well-defined cause of pain. For example, a patient with terminal cancer may experience pain but there is no expectation that the pain will go away by itself. The second is where there is no well-defined physical cause. This type of chronic pain carries the additional burden that it does not fit within a purely physiological model of pain, and many doctors are unwilling or unable to deal with pain from another perspective.

- Jim Pyke who had suffered for three years from intense back pain with apparently no cause said of his situation, 'There's nothing more discouraging than seeing a doctor after going through what I've gone through and then having him say, "Well, I've done my best, you're going to have to learn to live with it".'

In recent years pain clinics have been started which provide care and an often effective series of treatments for chronic pain sufferers, particularly those with no well-defined physical cause for their pain. Although nursing in a pain clinic is a specialism, the lessons about how pain clinics operate can be a useful guide when caring for patients who have less severe but nevertheless chronic pain such as lower back pain or pain from osteoarthritis.

In a pain clinic, it is usual to take a multi-dimensional approach to pain management, where several approaches are used simultaneously. Many of these treatments provide the patient with the feeling that he can exert some control over his pain. Discovering that pain is controllable is itself of immense benefit to pain sufferers.

Stress

Psychological factors are even more important in the control of chronic pain than acute pain. One of the major psychological factors is stress. Stress is a psychological and physiological state which arises from aversive events called stressors. The experience of stress is unpleasant and a nurse should aim to reduce a patient's stress as a way of reducing his suffering. In addition, however, stress is an important cause and enhancer of chronic pain, and its reduction should be used as a way of controlling such pain, breaking the vicious cycle of stress and pain.

Stressors

Stressors, as described above, are aversive events which can be either physiological or psychological and lead to stress. Typical physical stressors are:

- Excessive heat or cold
- Pathogens
- Tissue damage or severe burns
- Excessive noise
- Lack of food

Most people find the above stressful, though people find different physical stressors stressful to different degrees; some people get upset by noise, others by lack of food.

However, there is even more individual variation to psychological stressors. Whether an event is a psychological stressor or not depends on the interpretation put on it by the person. This means that a nurse cannot tell whether an event is stressful or not without asking the patient. Typical psychological stressors are:

- Bereavement and divorce
- Unemployment or redundancy
- A demanding job, children or elderly relative
- Lack of money
- Events which cause anger and frustration
- Being in pain and seeing others in pain

Stressors have physiological and psychological manifestations. The psychological manifestations are the feelings which are reported by someone who feels stressed, typically feelings of anxiety, depression, hopelessness and discomfort.

The main physiological manifestations are involuntary, i.e. they involve changes in body function over which there is normally no conscious control. These changes include:

- Changes in nervous activity: activation of the sympathetic nervous system and suppression of the parasympathetic nervous system
- Changes in blood chemistry: production of adrenaline, noradrenaline and cortico-steroids
- Changes in blood flow patterns: reduction in flow of blood to the periphery and stomach, and an increase in blood flow to muscles; increase in heart rate and blood pressure.

The physiological effects of stressors have a useful survival value: They prepare the body for 'fight or flight' at the approach of anything which is potentially harmful. However, if high stress levels occur over a period of time, stress hormones can have two major detrimental consequences.

First, corticosteroid stress hormones inhibit tissue recovery and are catabolic, i.e. they encourage tissue breakdown. Wound healing occurs fastest at night and adrenaline levels, which vary throughout the day, are lowest at night. Second, the stress hormones depress the activity of the immune system (see chapter 9) so the body is more vulnerable to infection.

A person's response to the occurrence of a stressor follows a predictable time course. First, there is an initial *alarm phase*, when the person reacts to the stress with lowered ability to cope. Second there is an *adaptation phase* when coping is optimal. Third, if the stressor persists, there is a *phase of exhaustion* when coping ability declines. Chronic pain sufferers may be in the phase of exhaustion: the pain has worn them out and they are not longer able to cope.

Selye (1956, 1976) suggests that, irrespective of the type of stressor, a person reacts to stress with a particular pattern of psychological and physiological manifestations which are unique to that person. This particular pattern is called the *general adaptation syndrome* or GAS. Some people develop gastric problems when stressed, some become irritable, some have headaches and some have back pain. Likewise for some people pain forms part of the GAS.

Stress increases pain experience and may actually be the cause of pain (e.g. tension headaches or stress-induced back pain). And pain is itself a stressor. Therefore, a major aim of pain control is to break the pain–stress cycle. Research (Keefe et al, 1987) shows that chronic pain sufferers who use stress- or pain-reducing strategies often find a considerable reduction in their experience of pain. Described below are some techniques for reducing chronic stress and chronic pain.

Relaxation

It is sometimes possible to achieve relaxation simply through suggestion or self-suggestion. In the previous section an example was given of a series of instructions which can help a person relax. By focusing attention on different parts of the body and consciously having a feeling of 'letting go', the patient can often achieve considerable relaxation.

Sometimes patients deny being tense when really they are. Simple feedback devices can help the patient when he is tense. For example, placing sellotape on a patient's forehead will indicate when the patient tenses his forehead muscles, which is often done under stress. Cold hands when in a warm room can mean that a person is stressed.

Biofeedback is a learning technique which tells the patient when he is tense. It involves taking electrical readings of body functions of which the person is not normally aware using an electrical biofeedback apparatus. The subject is presented with these readings and, by realising when he becomes more or less tense, uses them as a way of gaining control over functions which normally he cannot control. Of course, electrical sensors are not necessary for control of the autonomic nervous system: yogis have been found to be able to achieve similar effects through meditation. However, the biofeedback apparatus is a useful tool for someone who is not familar with meditation techniques.

The most commonly-used bodily functions for relaxation therapy are muscle tension (measured by an electromyogram or EMG) and peripheral skin temperature (measured by an electrical temperature probe). By learning how to reduce muscle tension or how to increase peripheral temperature (e.g. temperature of the finger) the patient learns to relax.

One important finding from research into biofeedback and, in particular, self-help schemes (Rosen, 1987) is that these techniques do not work well in the absence of a therapist. Some researchers question whether it is the biofeedback itself which is important for relaxation or whether it is the presence of a caring professional. Perhaps it is some combination of the two. Clearly, a good therapeutic relationship seems to help in any relaxation technique.

Massage is an under-rated but useful tool for relaxation. Massage to the forehead, back of the neck and base of the skull can be useful for people who suffer from headaches, as can massage to the shoulder muscles. Foot massage (massage to the sole of the foot) can have general relaxant properties. Massage is a technique which is easily taught to relatives. Spouses, in particular, often enjoy massaging their partner. The massage can involve the spouse in the care of the patient and, at the same time, improve the relationship.

The purpose of massage is to move and manipulate tissue, and not to rub the surface of the skin. The technique can be adjusted on the basis of the patient's perception that it is helping his pain.

Distraction

The experience of acute pain can often be modified by distraction, and a similar effect can be achieved for some patients with chronic pain. Patients can be taught self-distracting techniques, for example: 'When you feel a pain attack coming, try thinking about water flowing under a bridge'.

Research (Turk and Rudy, 1985) shows that when people focus attention on physical symptoms (e.g. gangrene spreading up the arm) or focus on their own inadequacy, their tolerance of pain is lowered. It can be suggested to patients that they focus their attention on positive aspects of the situation, and not think about negative characteristics of their bodies or personalities, as a way of controlling pain.

Change in life-style

Chronic pain sufferers find that the pain level varies over periods of time. Patients should be asked to establish what sort of situations increase their discomfort, so that, by avoiding these situations, they can minimise their pain. For example, if cold exacerbates the pain, the patient should try to keep warm. Patients often find that when they get angry, they experience more pain. By avoiding situations which lead to anger, discomfort can be reduced. The patient should be taught not to fight the stress in his life, but to try and avoid it.

Perceived control

The more that patients feel in control of their own lives and their pain, the less pain they experience. Training which teaches them to regain control often reduces the experience of pain. Indeed, all the techniques above have the effect of giving the patient the feeling that pain is not uncontrollable or unpredictable and to that extent they contribute to his feelings of self-determination and control. The belief that the patient can do something about his state is important for coping with long-term pain.

Physical treatments

Acupuncture and transcutaneous electrical nerve stimulation are both found to be of help for chronic pain sufferers, even though such techniques are effective only for short periods of time. However, by reducing pain even for a short period of time, the person becomes less stressed, and therefore more able to cope with pain. Physical treatments as well as drug treatments may reduce pain experience through expectancy effects.

Drug treatment

Peripherally-acting analgesics are a useful tool in the control of chronic pain but, except in the case of terminal illness, narcotic analgesics should not be used although they are sometimes, unwisely, prescribed for non-organic chronic pain. The main disadvantage of the narcotic analgesics is that adaptation to them occurs over a period of time so that the analgesic effect of the drug decreases. If prescribed a narcotic analgesic for an extended period, a pain sufferer may also become psychologically dependent on the drug, with the result that he expects and therefore experiences more pain if the drug is discontinued. Adjuvant analgesics are sometimes used for chronic pain relief but these should be restricted to antispasmodics, anticonvulsants and antidepressants. Sedative hypnotics and anxiolytic medications should not be used in the long-term management of chronic pain, except in the case of terminal illness, as they can lead to physical dependence as well as having unwanted side-effects (for more detail see Aronoff et al, 1986).

Overview of chronic pain management

There are physical and psychological techniques for controlling chronic pain. Both types of techniques are often used simultaneously in pain clinics. Compared with acute pain, however, psychological factors seem to play a more important role in the experience of chronic pain: psychological stressors cause stress and stress in turn causes pain.

The nurse has a particularly important role to play with chronic pain sufferers. First, she can act in an advisory capacity with regard to pain management and stress reduction. In so doing, she should develop a therapeutic relationship which may itself help the patient cope with pain. Second, the nurse should advise the patient on other forms of treatment, pain management or stress reduction clinics, for example.

When caring for a patient in chronic pain, it is easy to focus on the sufferer without paying attention to the relatives. However, chronic pain is not without consequences for the family: seeing a loved one in pain can be a psychological stressor for them too. Flor, Turk and Scholz (1987) found that the spouses of patients with chronic pain experienced more marital problems, distress and physical illness when compared with spouses of diabetics. Nursing patients with chronic pain requires more than a therapeutic relationship with the patient: the whole family may need such a relationship.

Someone suffering from chronic pain can be given the following advice.

1. Learn how to relax and how to avoid stress, as some people are able to control their pain through relaxation.

2. Find out what situations cause your pain to increase (e.g. overwork or cold) and avoid those situations.

3. Engage in positive rather than negative thinking, and use positive thinking to distract yourself from the pain.

4. Don't get angry, as this will just make you more stressed; learn to cope with, not to fight, your pain.

Finally, the nurse should realise that there is no magic cure for chronic pain, and that some patients suffer considerably because of it. The way she cares for them and the kind of therapeutic relationship she achieves can make pain much more bearable for her patients.

SUMMARY

The first part of this chapter covered the psychological and physiological interaction which leads to the perception of pain. Physical damage does not necessarily lead to the perception of pain, and pain can sometimes occur without physical damage. Patients with the same degree of physical damage can experience different levels of pain. The state of the pain receptors, the 'openness' of the gate in the spinal cord, the endorphin level in the brain, and the mood and attention level of the mind all influence the experience of pain.

The second part of this chapter covered acute pain management, first within the context of acute pain in an accident and emergency department and second in terms of preparation for postoperative pain. Various techniques were identified as helping relieve pain. For accident and emergency departments, the emphasis was on establishing a caring atmosphere, providing information and using distraction techniques. For preoperative preparation, the emphasis was placed on different types of information as well as on the importance of the therapeutic relationship between patient and nurse. Parents should be involved in both properative preparation and when their child is in casualty.

The third part of this chapter covered the management of chronic pain. Stress is an important contributor to chronic pain, so part of the management of chronic pain involves stress reduction.

Finally, it is important to emphasise that a patient who is reporting pain should not be dismissed as 'making a fuss'. The patient is in the best position to know how much pain he is feeling. Pain is a useful diagnostic indicator that something may be wrong, but even if no physical cause can be found, the experience of pain is not only distressing, but also profoundly affects a person's health and enjoyment of life.

References

Aronoff G M, Wagner J M and Spangler A S (1986) Chemical interventions for pain. *Journal of Consulting and Clinical Psychology,* **54**: 769–775.

Auerbach S M, Kendal P C, Cuttler H F and Levitt N R (1976) Anxiety, locus of control, type of preparatory information, and adjustment to dental surgery. *Journal of Consulting and Clinical Psychology,* **44**: 809–818.

Bandura A, O'Leary A, Taylor C B, Gauthier J and Gossard D (1987) Perceived self-efficacy and pain control: Opiod and nonopioid mechanisms. *Journal of Personality and Social Psychology,* **53**. 563–571.

Beales J G (1979) The effects of attention and distraction on pain among children attending a hospital casualty. In: *Research in Psychology and Medicine,* eds. Oborne D J, Guneberg M M and Eiser J R vol. 1, pp. 86–90. London: Academic Press.

Beales J G, Holt P L J, Keen J H and Melor V P (1983) Children with juvenile chronic arthritis: their beliefs about their illness and therapy. *Annals of the Rheumatic Diseases,* **42**: 481–486.

Beecher H K (1956) Relationship of significance of wound to the pain experienced. *Journal of American Medical Association*, **161**: 1609–1613.

Beecher H K (1957) The measurement of pain: prototype for the quantitative study of subjective responses. *Pharmacological Review*, **9**: 59–209.

Beutler L E, Engle D, Oro'-Beutler M E, Daldrup R and Meredith K (1986) Inability to express intense affect: a common link between depression and pain? *Journal of Consulting and Clinical Psychology*, **54**: 752–759.

Boore J R P (1978) *Prescription for Recovery*. RCN Research Series. London: Royal College of Nursing.

Brewster A B (1982) Chronically ill hospitalized children's concepts of their illness. *Pediatrics*, **69**: 355–362.

Camp L D and O'Sullivan P S (1987) Comparison of medical, surgical and oncology patients' descriptions of pain and nurses' documentation of pain assessments. *Journal of Advanced Nursing*, **12**: 593–598.

Cassell S and Paul M (1967) The role of puppet therapy on the emotional responses of children hospitalized for cardiac catheterization. *Pediatrics*, **71**: 233–239.

Egbert L D, Battit G E, Welch C E and Bartlett M K (1964) Reduction of postoperative pain by encouragement and instruction of patients. *New England Journal of Medicine*, **270**: 825–827,

Eiser C (1985) *The Psychology of Childhood Illness*. New York: Springer-Verlag.

Ferguson B F (1979) Preparing young children for hospitilization: a comparison of two methods. *Pediatrics*, **65**: 656–664.

Flaherty G G and Fitzpatrick J J (1978) Relaxation technique to increase comfort level of postoperative patients: a preliminary study. *Nursing Research*, **27**: 352–355.

Flor H, Turk D C and Scholz O B (1987) Impact of chronic pain on the spouse: marital, emotional and physical consequences. *Journal of Psychosomatic Research*, **31**: 63–71.

Kaplan R M, Metzger G and Jablecki C (1983) Brief cognitive and relaxation training increases tolerance for painful clinical electromyographic examination. *Psychosomatic Medicine*, **45**: 155–162.

Keefe F J, Caldwell D S, Queen K T, Gil K M, Martinex S, Croisson J E, Ogden W and Nunley J (1987) Pain coping stategies in osteoarthritis patients. *Journal of Consulting and Clinical Pschology*, **55**: 208–212.

Kirsch I (in press). *Changing Expectations: Expectancy Modification in Psychotherapy*. Chicago: Dorsey Press.

Langer E J, Janis I L and Wolfer J A (1975) Reduction of psychological stress in surgical patients. *Journal of Experimental Social Psychology*, **11**: 155–165.

Martelli M F, Auerbach S M, Alexander J and Mercuri L G (1987) Stress management in the health care setting: matching interventions with coping styles. *Journal of Consulting and Clinical Psychology*, **55**: 201–207.

McCaul K D and Macott J M (1984) Distraction and coping with pain. *Psychological Bulletin*, **95**: 516–533.

Melamed B G and Siegel L J (1975) Reduction of anxiety in children facing hospitalization and surgery by use of filmed modeling. *Journal of Consulting and Clinical Psychology*, **43**: 511–521.

Melamed B G, Meyer R, Gee C and Soule L (1976) The influence of time and type of preparation on children's adjustment to hospitalization. *Journal of Pediatric Psychology*, **1**: 31–37.

Melzack R (1975) The McGill Pain Qestionnaire: major properties and scoring methods. *Pain*, **1**: 277–299.

Melzack R and Wall P (1965) Pain mechanisms: a new theory. *Science*, **50**: 971–979.

Melzack R and Wall P (1968) Gate control theory of pain. In: *Pain*, eds. Soulairac A, Cahn J and Charpentior J, pp. 11–31. London: Academic Press.

Mogan J, Wells N and Robertson E (1985) Effects of preoperative teaching on postoperative pain: a replication and expansion. *International Journal of Nursing Studies*, **22**: 267–280.

Muller D J, Harris P J and Wattley L (1986) *Nursing Children: Psychology, Research and Practice*. London: Harper and Row.

Rodin J (1983) *Will This Hurt?* RCN Research Series. London: Royal College of Nursing.

Romano J M and Turner J A (1985) Chronic pain and depression: does the evidence support a relationship? *Psychological Bulletin,* **97**: 18–34.

Rosen G M (1987) Self-help treatment books and the commercialization of psychotherapy. *American Psychologist,* **42**: 46–51.

Ross D M and Ross S A (1984) Childhood pain: the school-aged child's viewpoint. *Pain,* **20**: 179–191.

Schwartz B H, Albino J E and Tedesco L A (1983) Effects of psychological preparation on children hospitalized for dental operations. *Journal of Pediatrics,* **102**: 634–638.

Selye H (1956) *The Stress of Life.* New York: McGraw-Hill.

Selye H (1976) *Stress in Health and Disease.* Sevenoaks: Butterworths.

Skipper J K and Leonard R C (1968) Children, stress and hospitalization: a field experiment. *Journal of Health and Social Behavior,* **9**: 275–281.

Taylor S E (1986) *Health Psychology.* New York: Landom House.

Turk D C and Rudy T E (1986) Assessment of cognitive factors in chronic pain: a worthwhile enterprise? *Journal of Consulting and Clinical Psychology,* **54**: 760–768.

Wallace L M (1986) Communication variables in the design of pre-surgical preparatory information. *British Journal of Clinical Psychology,* **25**: 111–118.

Weisenberg M (1980) Understanding pain phenomena. In: *Contributions to Medical Psychology,* ed. Rachman S, vol. 2, pp. 79–111. Oxford: Pergamon Press.

Wells J K, Howard G S, Nowlin W F and Vargas M J (1986) Presurgical anxiety and postsurgical pain and adjustment: effects of a stress inoculation procedure. *Journal of Consulting and Clinical Psychology,* **54**: 831–835.

Wilson-Barnett J and Fordham M (1982) *Recovery from Illness.* Chichester: John Wiley and Sons.

Wolfer J A and Visintainer M A (1979) Prehospital psychological preparation for tonsillectomy patients: effects on children's and parents' adjustment. *Pediatrics,* **64**: 646–655.

8

Caring for the Dying

and Bereaved

In popular fiction and drama, hospital staff often use the words, 'I'm sorry, there's nothing more we can do' to inform relatives of the impending death of a loved one. Such a comment implies that there is no point in providing care once the possibility of a cure has disappeared. The purpose of this chapter is to show that nothing could be further from the truth. People who are dying, people whose loved ones are dying and people who have been bereaved are usually in desperate need of both psychological and physical care. Nurses can help patients achieve a dignified death, and the care nurses give can help reduce the relatives' suffering caused by the death and their bereavement.

This chapter is divided into four sections.

1. Dying and death
2. Bereavement
3. Children's reactions to dying and bereavement
4. The nurse's perspective

The techniques discussed in this chapter build on the counselling and information-giving skills discussed in chapters 2 and 3.

DYING AND DEATH

Breaking the news

Should patients be told that they are dying, and if so how and when? Research shows that terminally-ill patients are often not told that they are dying yet more than 70 per cent of people report that they would want to be told if they were suffering from a condition which was likely to prove fatal (Carr, 1982).

Although almost 90 per cent of close relatives are told that their loved one is dying, this information is often kept from the patient. However, patients who are not told may guess that they are dying, and this can easily lead to communication between the patient and his relatives becoming strained. The patient and relatives can become involved in a 'hide-and-seek' game, with each one trying to hide his knowledge from the other and trying to guess what the other person knows. Such communication problems are likely to reduce the extent to which the patient and relatives are able to provide each other with emotional support at this difficult time.

The decision whether or not to tell the patient is typically taken by a doctor, who may also convey the information. Practice varies somewhat, and nurses can also make a contribution, either by advising the doctor or by being the most suitable person to break the news.

Several factors can affect whether and when a patient is told of impending death. First, the doctor or nurse needs to assess whether a patient wants to know his prognosis. A nurse is in a good position to make this assessment because she is often able to ask non-directive, exploratory questions (see chapter 2) without appearing unnatural. The answers to these can be used to find out what the patient knows about his condition and whether more information is needed. If the patient does want to know whether or not he is dying, the nurse may need to discuss this with a doctor before initiating action. However, a nurse should never dismiss a patient's questions with remarks like, 'You'll have to ask Dr Murray'. Instead, she should become actively involved in communicating with the doctor about the patient's wishes. Nurses can play a valuable role as 'advocates' for their patients though, if there is good communication between doctors and nurses and in particular if there is an agreed policy on communicating news about death, such advocacy should be unnecessary.

Relatives also affect the decision to tell a patient; they may advise that a patient should not be told when the patient himself wants to know. Counselling may be needed to convince relatives that the patient should be told about his condition. In some cases a nurse may be able to help relatives realise that the patient already suspects the truth. However, the nurse will be able to do this only if she has already used her communication skills to develop a therapeutic relationship with both the patient and his relatives.

Sometimes carers (doctors, nurses and relatives) prefer to hide the truth from a patient because they themselves find it stressful to talk to the patient about his death. However, from the patient's point of view there can be at least two advantages of knowing that he is going to die. The first is that guessing about death can itself be quite stressful, and some people find the uncertainty worse than the knowledge of death. The second is that a person can then make final arrangements so that he can die a dignified death knowing that his affairs are in order.

People have different ways of coping with death, just as people have different ways of coping with pain (see chapter 7). For example, people who have a high need for control and who typically react to stress and pain by seeking information are likely to want to know about their impending death. On the other hand, patients who typically respond to stress by distraction and withdrawal may prefer not to know. The patient should be allowed to choose his own way of coping with his death.

The best person to tell a patient that he is dying is someone who has developed a good therapeutic relationship with him. A nurse breaking the news will need to select her moment carefully. She will need time to break the news, and time to let the information sink in. She may also need time simply to sit with the patient and hold his hand. Breaking such news can be stressful to the nurse giving the news, but it is a crucially important part of giving care.

Reactions to the news of terminal illness

Kubler-Ross (1969) suggests that the reaction to the knowledge that one is terminally ill typically goes through five stages: denial, anger, bargaining, depression and acceptance. Subsequent writers (Schulz and Aderman, 1974; Kastenbaum and Weisman, 1972) point out that these stages do not always occur, and that they do not necessarily occur in this sequence. Furthermore, it has been shown (Carr, 1982; Taylor, 1986) that fear and anxiety are also experienced by people who know that they are dying. However, Kubler-Ross' stages, with the addition of fear and anxiety, provide a good picture of the dying patient's experiences.

Fear and anxiety

One reaction which people who are terminally ill have is the feeling of fear. This can consist of:

1. Fear of pain and suffering

2. Fear of loneliness and of dying alone

3. Fear for their relatives and how they will cope with the situation

4. Fear of what will happen after death

A nurse should provide the patient with opportunities to ask questions in relation to these different fears, and some measure of reassurance is possible. For example, the patient can be told that analgesics will be available to take away the pain. The nurse should emphasise that full care is given up to the point of death; some patients fear that they will not be cared for if labelled a 'hopeless case'. Assurances about the nurse's presence can help allay the fear of extreme loneliness that some patients experience. Presencing (i.e. the nurse simply being with the patient, see chapter 2) is a valuable part of caring for the dying. The patient can also be told that most deaths are painless, and that the patient just slips away to whatever he believes comes next.

If a patient is worried about how relatives will cope, the best people to provide reassurance are usually the relatives themselves. Depending on the circumstances it may be possible to have a word with the family to see if there is some way the patient can be comforted in this respect. Patients' worries about their relatives span the time after, as well as the period leading up to, death.

A dying person is often worried about what appear to the nurse to be trivial concerns, such as who will feed the budgie or who will return a library book. From the patient's perspective, these are not trivial, and practical help from the nurse to sort out the undone odds and ends may reduce anxiety and enhance the dignity of dying.

In general, younger patients (under the age of 50) are more likely to be anxious than older patients (Hinton, 1972), but patients of all ages may experience worry of one form or another.

Caring for terminally-ill people with anxieties is similar to caring for other people who are anxious. The nurse must first show that she accepts the anxiety before attempting to provide reassurance. And when the nurse feels that it is time to provide reassurance it should be specific, practical and realistic, rather than simply exhorting the patient to cheer up and stop worrying.

- Mrs Anderson knew that she was suffering from an incurable form of cancer. She confided in a nurse that she was worried about how her husband would cope with running the home and looking after their young daughter as his domestic skills were very limited. The nurse tried to reassure Mrs Anderson by saying, 'Don't you worry yourself about that. I'm sure he'll get along fine'. However, this did not lessen Mrs Anderson's anxiety, so a few days later she expressed similar anxieties to another nurse. This nurse showed that she accepted Mrs Anderson's anxiety as reasonable by saying, 'Yes, that must be very worrying for you'. Furthermore, through talking to Mrs Anderson's relatives, the nurse had already learned that Mr Anderson's mother had agreed to help around the house and had started giving him cookery lessons. The relatives had not mentioned this to Mrs Anderson because they were afraid that it might upset her. In fact, she was very relieved when the nurse told her about the family's plans.

Denial

Some patients do not react initially with fear and anxiety. Instead, they deny the prognosis: they may tell the hospital staff that they have got it wrong. The nurse could reply, 'I hope that we are wrong' or 'We can pray that you will get better' but should not deny the diagnosis. It is worth remembering, too, that diagnoses of death can be wrong. If the patient is clinging to hope, that hope should not be destroyed. The patient may need time for the news to sink in and may ask the same question again and again. Some patients only accept that they are dying when their physical condition deteriorates markedly.

Anger

A terminally-ill patient may become angry: angry that this is happening to him and that it is his life which is being disrupted, and angry with other people such as nurses, doctors and relatives. The best way to react to the anger is to listen, remembering that any hurtful things the patient says are the result of his extreme suffering. It is not advisable to say, 'I understand how you must be feeling' because this will sound false and patronising. Instead exploratory statements like, 'I think you are angry with me' or 'Do you feel angry about this?' can be used. Nor will it help to explain to the patient that he has it all wrong. The patient is not being rational, and needs time to work through his anger. The nurse may also need to explain to relatives that the patient's anger towards them is a normal reaction to learning of one's death.

Bargaining

The patient may try to bargain instead of getting angry, as a way of fighting the news of death. An uncharacteristic amount of charitable or good behaviour (e.g. meticulously following doctor's orders) may indicate that the patient is striking a bargain to save himself. Sometimes the patient makes a pact with God about what he will do if he is spared. Bargaining is based on an implicit feeling that the world is just.

Depression

Some patients go through a phase of depression. They are unhappy because of the loss of physical strength which has already occurred, and the loss of the future life which is now denied them. Under such circumstances, the patient experiences psychological suffering and appears inactive and sad. Kubler-Ross refers to the stage of depression as a time for 'anticipatory grief'. The stage of depression, although unpleasant, may have the psychological function of preparing the patient for what is to come. As such, Kubler-Ross suggests that the depression should not be countered but be allowed to run its course.

Acceptance

At this final stage, the patient is no longer angry or depressed. Instead, he accepts the prospect of his death in a calm, peaceful and dignified way. He is likely to want to withdraw more and more from what is going on around him, and may concentrate his thoughts on the past and want to think about the good times in his life. He may appreciate non-verbal contact more than talking, and in particular will appreciate the presence of loved ones.

Acceptance is more likely if the patient is able to have a positive evaluation of his life. Talking with him about what he has done is one way to help a patient see his life in perspective as being good. Acceptance can also be helped if people have religious beliefs that life is not ended by death. Many religions suggest an after-death experience, and patients may wish to speak to a priest or other religious leader during the period leading up to their death. Even if patients do not have strong religious feelings, they can still believe that they have achieved 'symbolic immortality', either in terms of their children, or in terms of the useful work they have done during their life.

A nurse should recognise and help the patient's striving towards acceptance and his need to find meaning in his life. Not only should the nurse talk (and enable others to talk) about the patient's life, but she should also allow the patient to talk about the past in terms of what he has achieved, thereby enhancing the sense of permanency and purpose.

Caring for the relatives

When nursing terminally-ill patients, it is essential to cater for relatives' as well as patients' needs. If relatives wish to participate in providing physical care for the terminally-ill patient they should be encouraged to do so, since this can help reduce any feelings of guilt once they are bereaved. However, relatives should not be made to feel guilty if they are unable or unwilling to participate in the patient's physical care, and they should certainly not be made to feel that it is their duty to take full responsibility for the patient's care. Even if relatives are not actively participating in providing physical assistance, it is important to involve them by communicating with them about the patient's care. Relatives can also play a vital role by providing emotional support.

Irrespective of the extent to which they are involved in looking after the patient, relatives and other loved ones are likely to require emotional support themselves. This support may be provided by a variety of people, such as the following.

1. *The patient*: Sometimes a patient and a relative are able to offer emotional support to one another. To facilitate this, patients and their relatives should be given the opportunity to be together without interruption and with as much privacy as possible. The patient remains part of a family while dying and, because the period of dying focuses attention on the important things in life, it can be a time when relationships are restated and strengthened.

2. *Relatives of other patients*: Relatives can find it helpful to share experiences with other people who are in a similar position so it is a good idea to introduce them to one another. Also, it is useful if somewhere can be provided for them to chat over coffee. At the very least, the nurse should ensure that relatives know how to find the nearest refreshment facilities.

3. *Nurses*: A nurse should always find time to speak to relatives. It is important not to restrict conversation to the patient's needs, but to encourage relatives to talk about their own needs and feelings. Some relatives try to forget their own needs because they perceive the patient's needs to be more pressing. For example, relatives may be exhausted by being constantly at the bedside. Under such circumstances a nurse can suggest that the relative has a rest, but suggest it in a way which is focused on the patient, for example, 'Why don't you go home for a little while. That way you will be stronger to talk to your husband later on this evening when he will be more awake. And of course, we will telephone immediately if any change takes place'.

Close relatives will usually want to be with the patient when he dies. Therefore it is important to find out whether this is so and how relatives can be contacted quickly.

The period surrounding death

Death itself can take many different forms. Sometimes the patient is in a state of acceptance and dies with loving relatives. In other cases the patient dies struggling to survive. It is important for nurses, relatives and patients not to have preconceived ideas about what death ought to be.

Dying is one of the most private and intimate times of a patient's life. If relatives are present, the nurse may have to consider whether or not she should intrude on such an intimate family situation. However, if a nurse has formed a good therapeutic relationship with the patient and relatives they may wish her to be there and lend her support by her mere presence.

If relatives are not present, then the nurse may wish to be with the patient during his death. Many patients become quite confused or even unconscious during the moments leading up to death, but a caring presence can be a very great comfort.

Irrespective of the circumstances in which a patient dies, news of the death will usually come as a great shock to the patient's relatives. This is so even in cases where the relatives knew that the patient was terminally ill. Although there is no easy way of telling people that a loved one has died, there are ways for the nurse to show relatives that she cares about them and about their loss. News of a patient's death should be broken to relatives in a quiet place where they can have privacy. As with any unpleasant news, relatives should, if possible, be seated when the information is given. If the information is given over the telephone it should not be given too abruptly. Instead, the listener should be given the opportunity to guess the news before it is broken, for example:

● Hello, Mrs Smith, it's Sister Burton here. I am afraid I have got some bad news for you (*pause*). Your mother (*pause*) passed away peacefully a few minutes ago.

The nurse who breaks the news in person should speak calmly but should try to express empathy, for example, by placing her hand on the bereaved person's hand or shoulder. A nurse should offer to sit with the relatives after they have been given the news; this is particularly important if only one relative is present. She should not feel that she has to keep talking to the bereaved person all the time she is with him. Comfort and support can be provided just by being there.

While getting over the immediate shock of the death of a loved one, some relatives are unable to make simple decisions. It is at this stage that simple, practical suggestions can be found very helpful, for example suggestions about death certificates and funerals. Other relatives are less debilitated by the death, and may wish to ask questions. Religions typically have rituals and beliefs associated with death, and the nurse should be sensitive in finding out about and respecting the religious beliefs and customs of patients and relatives. Even people who do not normally practise a religion may prefer a particular religious ceremony at a time of death. Neuberger (1987) provides a useful summary of the different practices relating to death which are adopted by the major religions.

The bereaved person should be asked if there is another relative or friend whom he would like to be with and, if so, staff should try to contact this person. The nurse should also check how the bereaved person is getting home, and what support if any can be arranged at home.

If relatives are not present at the death, they may wish to see the patient's body, and should be given every opportunity to do so. The term 'body' should, however, not be used; instead one can say for example, 'Would you like to see your husband now?' Care should be taken so that the viewing of the body is dignified; thought should be given to the location and presentation of the body, and the bereaved relative should be warned if there are any disfigurements.

Some relatives are so numb with shock that they do not know whether or not they want to see the body. As viewing the body can be an important first stage in the grieving process, the nurse can make a slight suggestion to the effect that, 'Some people find afterwards that they were pleased they saw their husband, but some prefer not to'. Such suggestions should be very tentative as the nurse's aim is to try and find out the relative's real wishes during this period of shock.

It is important to create an atmosphere in which bereaved people feel able to express their feelings and to weep. Similarly, the nurse should not feel embarrassed about shedding a few tears herself. If she has developed a relationship with a patient, it is natural for her, too, to feel sad when he dies, and her tears will tell the bereaved that she cared for their loved one and shares their grief.

BEREAVEMENT

Whether a nurse is working in the community or in a hospital, she is likely to meet people who are still experiencing the effects of bereavement. She should be prepared to provide support for any bereaved person, not just for those who have been newly bereaved.

Reactions to bereavement

Like reactions to terminal illness, reactions to bereavement vary from person to person, but can be described in terms of a 'typical' sequence of stages. For example, Carr (1982) outlines three phases of grief.

1. *Numbness and disbelief*: Especially if the death has occurred unexpectedly, the bereaved person may initially react with feelings of numbness and disbelief. This phase can last for anything from a few minutes to a few weeks.

2. *Acute grief*: Once the bereaved person becomes aware of the reality of the loss, he will usually experience overwhelming anguish and despair, and will be preoccupied with thoughts of the person who has died. The duration of the acute grief phase varies considerably from person to person, but it is typically between three and 10 weeks.

3. *Recovery*: During this phase, the bereaved person gradually adjusts to his loss and to life without the person who has died. This process of reconstruction usually takes between six and 18 weeks.

These three phases are not clear cut. The experiences which characterise a particular phase become less frequent but do not totally disappear when the bereaved person progresses to the next phase. For example, people who have begun to recover from their grief may still, on occasions, experience feelings of disbelief or anguish.

Most people's reactions to bereavement (especially during the acute grief phase) involve a complex mixture of psychological and physical experiences. The precise nature of this mixture varies according to the individual.

Psychological aspects of grief

Grief often includes such emotions as sadness, anger, anxiety, guilt, loneliness, helplessness and relief. Bereaved people sometimes find their feelings of anger and relief particularly puzzling and difficult to handle. For instance, they may feel angry with the dead person for having left them to cope alone, but at the same time they may feel guilty about being angry with someone who has died. Feelings of relief are particularly likely to arise when the death has occurred after a prolonged illness. Relatives may feel relieved that the patient's suffering has ended and that they no longer have to carry the burden of caring for him. Again, such feelings can make the bereaved person feel guilty. The bereaved person should be encouraged to express his feelings and be helped to regard them as reasonable.

During the acute phase of grief, it is common for people to be preoccupied with memories of the person who has died. As a result, the bereaved person is likely to have difficulty in concentrating and may behave absent-mindedly. Sometimes, he will also experience hallucinations, thinking that he has seen or heard the deceased person. Some bereaved people want to avoid any reminders of the person who has died, whereas others cling on to things which remind them of their loved one.

Physical aspects of grief

It is common for bereaved people to have difficulty sleeping and eating. They may also experience various physical sensations, such as tightness in the throat or chest, breathlessness, hollowness in the stomach, a dry mouth, weakness and lack of energy (Worden, 1982). It is not uncommon for the bereaved to have physical symptoms which mimic those previously experienced by the person who has died. Although the various physical aspects of grief have a strong psychological basis, it is important to realise that they have a real physical effect. Thus, a bereaved person should not be told that his physical symptoms are 'all in the mind'. Physical and psychological processes influence one another in a variety of complex ways (see chapter 9).

Bereaved people are more at risk than other people of becoming ill (Maddison and Viola, 1968) and of dying (Parkes, Benjamin and Fitzgerald, 1969; Jones, 1987). The risk of death is greatest for widowers during the first six months after their wife's death (Clayton, 1979).

Caring for the bereaved

What bereaved people usually need most is to be allowed time to grieve. It is important to appreciate that grief is a normal, necessary process and does not disappear soon after the funeral. Grief is not a disease, so one should not try to provide an instant cure. However, the nurse can help people to cope with their grief by showing them that she cares about their loss and is willing to offer support.

Worden (1982) has identified four 'tasks of mourning', and he argues that accomplishing these tasks is essential to the bereaved person's future psychological well-being. These tasks provide a useful framework for considering the ways in which support and care can be provided.

Accepting the reality of the loss

In order to grieve, bereaved people need to accept that the deceased person is really dead; they need to let the implications of the news sink in. One of the main ways in which people can come to accept the reality of their loss is by talking about what has happened. Many bereaved people feel the need to talk through the circumstances surrounding the death again and again. The nurse can help by encouraging them to talk and by being a patient listener. She should accept this as a normal part of grieving, and should avoid making comments like, 'You told me all that yesterday'. The bereaved person may be reluctant to talk to other relatives about the death for fear of adding to their distress. The nurse, as someone who is less personally involved, can play an important role by listening.

Experiencing the pain of grief

The second task of mourning is to experience the pain of grief. Research has shown that if a person tries to avoid or suppress the pain of bereavement, he is likely to encounter psychological problems at a later stage in life, for instance, he may show a very severe reaction to a subsequent loss (Hollingsworth and Pasnau, 1977). The pain of grief consists of the various psychological and physical reactions described earlier. Bereaved people can be helped to experience this pain by being encouraged to talk about how they are feeling, both emotionally and physically. Also, the carer should not continually try to cheer them up, but should show acceptance when they express their feelings through, for example, weeping.

Adjusting to life without the deceased

The death of a close relative or friend usually necessitates some adjustments to the person's way of life. The precise nature of these adjustments will depend on the type of relationship which existed between the bereaved and the deceased. Adjustments which bereaved people may have to make include coming to terms with living alone, bringing up children alone instead of with a partner, acquiring new skills and taking on new responsibilities. The nurse can aid people in accomplishing this task of mourning by discussing practical issues, offering advice about how they might set about acquiring new skills and informing them about support groups available locally (such as 'Cruse', which is a support group for widows, widowers and their families). It is also a good idea for the nurse to express confidence in the bereaved person's ability to acquire new skills and take on new responsibilities.

Withdrawing and reinvesting emotional energy

This final task of mourning is a particularly difficult one and is often not successfully accomplished (Worden, 1982). It involves the bereaved person withdrawing emotional energy from the process of mourning, and using it to develop existing or new relationships with people who are still alive. Once a person is ready to face this final task of mourning, he should be helped to appreciate that a new relationship is not a replacement for his relationship with the person who has died, since every relationship is unique.

CHILDREN'S REACTIONS TO DYING AND BEREAVEMENT

In order to provide appropriate care for children who are dying or who have been bereaved, the nurse needs to appreciate that the way children understand and react to death changes with age. This section outlines these developmental changes.

Up to seven months old

Children do not form strong attachments with particular people until they are about seven months old (see chapter 6). Therefore, children below this age do not usually show any obvious reaction to the death of a familiar person, so long as they continue to receive good physical and psychological care.

Seven months to two years old

If a child in this age group has formed an attachment to a particular person, his reaction to the death of that person will typically be similar to his reaction to more temporary separations. Thus, he may show distress in the form of protest, despair and detachment (see chapter 6). The young child's distress can be reduced by the presence of other people with whom he has a good relationship.

Two to five years old

From the age of about two years, children begin to talk about death. However, words like 'dead' and 'died' do not mean the same to a young child as they do to an adult. For instance, two- to five-year-olds usually talk about death as if it were reversible; in other words, they view it as temporary rather than final. They regard dying as similar to going to sleep or going on a journey. As with the previous age group, two- to five-year-olds' reactions to bereavement consist mainly of separation anxiety. A young child whose mother has died may be frightened about being left alone with no one to look after him. Such anxieties can be reduced by assuring bereaved children that they will be cared for. As soon as specific arrangements have been made regarding the care of a bereaved child, these should be explained to him.

Five to nine years old

Children in this age group are becoming increasingly aware that death is much more serious than other separations or departures. From about the age of five, children usually know that death is final and irreversible. Some children in this age group also realise that death is universal, that is they know it will happen to everyone including themselves. However, other children do not seem to regard death as universal, and their ideas about death are sometimes heavily influenced by fantasy. Not surprisingly, the children who are most likely to have a realistic view of death are those who have lost a close relative or friend (Reilly, Hasazi and Bond, 1983) and those who are terminally ill (Waechter, 1971).

   Since five- to nine-year-olds realise that death is serious, their reactions to bereavement and terminal illness can be severe. However, these reactions sometimes take a different form from those of adults. There are two main reasons for this. First, the child may not yet have achieved as complete an understanding of death as an adult has. Second, the child will be less able to use language as a tool for expressing and coming to terms with his reaction to death.

   Bereaved children, like bereaved adults, sometimes experience feelings of guilt. Children's guilt can be particularly severe because they have less understanding than adults about the causes of death and, in particular, they may believe that their own naughtiness has caused the death of a loved one. It is, therefore, important to give bereaved children realistic explanations of why someone has died.

   Anger is another grief reaction which is common to both children and adults. While bereaved adults usually express their anger verbally, bereaved children will often express it through bad behaviour, such as temper tantrums or disobedience. It is useful if those who are looking after a bereaved child can be prepared for the fact that a child's grief does not always take the same form as an adult's.

   From the age of about six years, children who are terminally ill typically realise that their illness is serious and this often results in them experiencing anxiety (Spinetta, 1974). In some cases, terminally-ill children directly express their anxiety about death (Waechter, 1971). In other cases, the child expresses more general anxiety and does not specifically mention death, but even this more general anxiety probably indicates that the child is aware of the seriousness of his condition. Spinetta, Rigler and Karon (1973) found that six- to 10-year-old children who were terminally ill showed more anxiety than those who were suffering from a chronic but non-fatal illness. This was the case despite the fact that none of the terminally-ill children had been told their prognosis. Thus, it is clearly very difficult (if not impossible) to protect children from the knowledge that they are dying. Children are able to work out a great deal from non-verbal cues and from their parents' reactions. As with adults, it is important to give children the opportunity to express their anxieties. Children may find it easier to express their anxieties through play, drawing or talking about pictures, rather than through a purely verbal conversation. The child's anxieties should be accepted as legitimate but, at the same time, it will usually be possible to offer some form of reassurance, for example that the child's parents will be with him when he dies.

Over nine years old

By the age of about nine or 10 years, most children have developed an understanding of death which is very similar to an adult's. Also, as children approach adolescence, their reactions to bereavement and terminal illness become increasingly adult-like, so many of the points which were made about helping adults cope with dying and bereavement can be applied to children in this older age group. On the other hand, it should be remembered that teenagers are not the same as adults. For example, they are less likely to have had previous experience of grief. Also, despite their apparent independence, many teenagers are in fact very emotionally dependent on their parents, which must be remembered if it is the parent who has died.

The stages which have been outlined above provide an approximate guide to the ideas and reactions which are most likely to occur at a particular age. But, as with other aspects of child development, each child is unique and develops at his own rate, so it is important to assess the needs of the individual child.

Communicating with terminally-ill children about death

Terminally-ill children often realise that they are dying from events around them. Shielding a child from talk about death may not be in the child's best interest as children can develop upsetting fantasies about death. If the child is allowed to talk about death these fantasies can be brought into the open.

Researchers who work with dying children (Bluebond-Langer, 1977) recommend that children, like adults, should be given honest answers about death. As with any form of counselling, what is said to a child should be determined by what the child himself says. The child may give information or ask questions directly, but often the child will seek answers through hidden questions. Extreme sensitivity is needed in uncovering what a child knows, what he wants to know and what he is able to understand.

Death can sometimes best be explained by examples which draw on the child's previous experience, for instance by reference to the death of a pet. Some children gain relief from the knowledge that, although they will be dead, their parents and friends will still be living and thinking about them. Children may also gain relief from the knowledge that their parents will be with them when they die.

As parents may have been the major source of personal information in the past, it is often best to involve parents in talking to a child about the child's death. However, the nurse will have to ascertain first how the parents relate to the child and how they are coping with their own distress. For example, parents who are avoiding the child's questions and who are made anxious by them may need time to come to terms with the prospect of their child's death themselves before they are able to communicate effectively with him. Under such circumstances, the nurse's task is to help parents to appreciate the importance of dealing openly with their child's questions about death.

Terminally-ill children

Terminally-ill children have many of the same needs as other children. In particular, they need to play and to have fun. In some American hospitals clowns and other entertainers are employed to help fulfil this basic childhood need. But even if professional entertainers are not available, nurses and parents can help make the child's remaining days as happy as possible.

The siblings of terminally-ill children often have difficulties in adjusting to the situation. The parents' attention is focused away from the healthy siblings during a terminal illness and, not surprisingly, emotional and behavioural problems can occur as a consequence. A nurse can help by acknowledging siblings and also by involving them during visiting times in play activities on the ward. A terminally-ill child, like any other patient, remains part of a family.

The bereaved child

Many of the points discussed above in relation to terminally-ill children can also be applied when communicating with children who have a terminally-ill relative or who have been bereaved.

Again, it is best to deal openly with the child's questions about death and to encourage him to talk about his anxieties and other emotions. Young children sometimes blame themselves for the death of a loved one; for example, they may believe that Mummy died because they were naughty. Adults can reduce such feelings of guilt by helping children understand the circumstances surrounding the death. Bereaved children, like bereaved adults, may find that talking about the circumstances surrounding the death helps them to accept the reality of their loss. Visiting the graveside can also be helpful in this respect. As with terminally-ill children, the child's own questions and comments will often provide the best guide to what the child should be told.

The most appropriate person to talk to a child about the death of a loved one is someone who already has a good therapeutic relationship with the child, such as a parent or another relative. However, this person will probably be having to cope with his own grief. Here a nurse can make a valuable contribution by providing emotional support and by helping adults to appreciate the importance of communicating openly with children about death.

THE NURSE'S PERSPECTIVE

The task of helping terminally-ill patients and their families to cope with strong emotions and unpleasant experiences can be stressful and emotionally demanding for the nurse.

For the nurse at the start of her career who has probably had little prior experience of death, the task of caring for the terminally ill has the additional burden of novelty. In British culture death is a 'taboo' subject, and the student nurse needs to adjust to working in a previously unmentionable area. Worries about 'knowing what to say' are common, but it is actually not necessary to say very much. What is necessary is the ability to listen and understand.

For the more experienced nurse, caring for the terminally ill still remains one of the most demanding areas of nursing. It is important for the provision of good care that nurses recognise their own psychological need for support. Without support the nurse may suffer from 'burnout', a feeling of emotional exhaustion, numbness and detachment.

Some hospitals run mentor schemes or staff support groups. If these formal support facilities are available, it is beneficial to participate actively in them, as good care of patients is based on good care of nurses. If organised schemes are not available, it is possible to obtain support more informally by sharing feelings and experiences with a friend. The ability to seek and accept support is not a sign of weaknes, but is a sign of appreciating the importance of maintaining one's strength.

There are two purposes of a formal or informal support group. The first is to allow nurses to share their feelings and experiences. The second is to provide a forum for demonstrating that life goes on despite the death of many patients. It is crucial that nurses provide each other with support in this way.

SUMMARY

This chapter covers the topic of dying and bereavement, and develops further the skills of counselling and information-giving described in chapters 2 and 3. The chapter is in four sections: dying and death, bereavement, children's reactions to dying and bereavement and the nurse's perspective.

There are several types of reaction to the knowledge of one's death (fear, anxiety, denial, anger, bargaining, depression and acceptance, for instance) and each form of reaction requires a different type of care. Relatives can play a crucial role in caring for the dying, and need special care both before and after the patient's death. In both dying and bereavement, the process of adjusting to loss is usually a lengthy one.

Children's knowledge of death varies according to age and the individual child. Communication with children about death should be based on the particular child's knowledge and ability to understand.

Caring for the terminally ill is a particularly stressful aspect of nursing, so the nurse should be prepared both to accept support from other nurses and to provide support for them.

Finally it should be re-emphasised that the need for psychological care does not disappear when a patient is terminally ill or when he dies. If anything, the importance of psychological care increases in such circumstances.

References

Bluebond-Langer M (1977) Meanings of death in children. In: *New meanings of Death*, ed. Feifel H. New York: McGraw-Hill.

Carr A T (1982) Dying and bereavement. In: *Psychology for Nurses and Health Visitors*, ed. Hall J. London: Macmillan.

Clayton P J (1979) The sequelae and nonsequelae of conjugal bereavement. *Psychiatry*, **136**: 1530–1534.

Hinton J (1972) *Dying*. Harmondsworth: Penguin.

Hollingsworth C E and Pasnau R O (1977) Delayed grief and pathological mourning. In: *The Family in Mourning: A Guide for Health Professionals*, eds. Hollingsworth C E and Pasnau R O. New York: Grune and Stratton.

Jones D R (1987) Heart disease mortality following widowhood: some results from the OPCS longitudinal study. *Journal of Psychosomatic Research*, **32**: 325–333.

Kastenbaum R and Weisman A D (1972) The psychological autopsy as a research procedure in gerontology. In: *Research Planning and Action for the Elderly*, eds. Kent D P, Kastenbaum R and Sherwood S. New York: Behavioral Publications.

Kubler-Ross E (1969) *On Death and Dying*. London: Tavistock Publications.

Maddison D C and Viola A (1968) The health of widows in the year following bereavement. *Journal of Psychosomatic Research*, **12**: 297–306.

Neuberger J (1987) *Caring for Dying People of Different Faiths*. London: Austen Cornish.

Parkes C M, Benjamin B and Fitzgerald R G (1969) Broken heart: a statistical study of increased mortality among widowers. *British Medical Journal*, **i**: 740–743.

Reilly T P, Hasazi J E and Bond L A (1983) Children's conceptions of death and personal mortality. *Journal of Pediatric Psychology*, **8**: 21–31.

Schulz R and Aderman D (1974) Clinical research and the stages of dying. *Omega*, **5**: 137–143.

Spinetta J J, (1974) The dying child's awareness of death: a review. *Psychological Bulletin*, **81**: 256–260.

Spinetta J J, Rigler D and Karon M (1973) Anxiety in the dying child. *Pediatrics*, **52**: 841–845.

Taylor S E (1986) *Health Psychology*. New York: Random House.

Waechter E (1971) Children's awareness of fatal illness. *American Journal of Nursing*, **71**: 1168–1172.

Worden J W (1982) *Grief Counselling and Grief Therapy*. London: Tavistock Publications.

9
Mind and Body

The idea that state of mind affects physical illness has been with us for many years. Two thousand years ago the Roman physician, Galen, believed that 'melancholic' (i.e. sad) women were at greater risk of cancer than 'sanguine' (i.e. hopeful and confident) women. This assumed relationship between psychology and physical illness remained up to the beginning of the twentieth century, when rapid developments in the physical treatment of illness led to the belief that illness was a purely biological phenomenon.

Galen's assumption was not based on any scientific evidence. Recent research, however, has demonstrated the importance of psychological factors in physical illness. Interestingly, Galen's suggestion that 'melancholic' women are more at risk of cancer has received scientific support (Lambley, 1986).

Today, the purely biological model of disease based on the concept of 'one germ, one disease, one therapy' is seen as too simplistic (Engel, 1977). Baker (1987) concludes, 'Psychological factors probably can affect the outcome of virtually every disease'.

The aim of this chapter is to enable the nurse to anticipate illness on the basis of the psychological characteristics of the patient and so to take preventative action, to encourage psychological states which facilitate the patient's recovery, and to educate people who are well so as to maintain their good health.

This chapter provides an account of the psychology of certain diseases and is divided into three sections. The first section explains how psychological factors affect the immune system, the second section deals with psychological factors related to cancer and the final section examines the role played by psychological factors in coronary heart disease. There are, in fact, many other illnesses where psychological factors play a role: rheumatoid arthritis, asthma, migraine, gastric ulcers and ulcerative colitis are all thought to have some psychological basis though these illnesses will not be considered in this chapter. However, there is some commonality between the psychology of different illnesses. Friedman and Booth-Kewley (1987) provide evidence for a 'disease-prone personality', a type of personality which leads to the risk of a variety of different illnesses. The disease-prone personality includes the traits of anxiety, depression and anger.

Although this chapter focuses on the relation between the mind and physical illness, this theme has already appeared in some earlier chapters. For example, preoperative preparation has been shown to lead to faster recovery after surgery (see chapter 7), and an increase in perceived control in long-stay hospitalised elderly patients decreases their mortality and morbidity (see chapters 1 and 5).

THE IMMUNE SYSTEM

The immune system is the body's own surveillance mechanism whose main function is to destroy bacteria, viruses and cancerous tissue. In addition, the immune system regulates susceptibility to allergies, and is also responsible for autoimmune disorders in which the immune cells attack the normal tissues of the body. The effectiveness of the immune system is important to the prevention and cure of a wide range of different illnesses.

The immune system is composed of a number of different components. First, there are lymphocytic cells, of which there are two sorts: *T lymphocytes*, produced in the bone marrow and processed by the thymus, and *B lymphocytes* produced by and maturing in the bone marrow. The lymphocytes engulf and destroy bacteria and viruses as well as producing antibodies which coat the surfaces of bacteria and other foreign bodies to neutralise them and make them easier to 'consume'. The less active the lymphocytes, the more a person is likely to become infected.

In addition to the lymphocytes, there are a number of other immune cells which increase or suppress the activity of the lymphocytes, or have an immune function of their own. These include *helper T* and *suppressor T cells*, *mast cells*, *macrophages* and *natural killer cells*. The latter have an important role in preventing cancer. Also, the substance interferon produced by the immune system plays a role in inhibiting the action of viruses. Our current state of knowledge is such that we do not know precisely how the different aspects of the immune system work together; for example, the activity of the different components of the immune system can vary independently. However, it is known that psychological factors can affect the different components separately as well as the general effectiveness of the immune system as a whole. The overall effectiveness of the immune system is referred to as the *level of immunocompetence*. A body with a high level of immunocompetence is better able to fight infection than one with a low level of immunocompetence.

Psychoimmunology

One of the earliest studies in psychoimmunology was carried out early this century by the researcher Ishigami (1919) who examined lymphocyte activity in patients with chronic tuberculosis. Ishigami found that the activity of the lymphocytes decreased during periods of emotional excitement, and suggested that the 'stress of contemporary life' could impair the functioning of the immune system.

Other researchers (reviewed in Jemmott and Locke, 1984) have found that stressful life events precede many other sorts of physical illness, including respiratory infections such as colds. Colds are not just caused by the presence of a cold virus; after all, cold viruses are often present in the air and people frequently inhale them, yet do not always catch a cold. Although a cold virus is necessary for catching such an infection, it is not the only factor involved. A person's immune system must be functioning less well than normal so that the virus gets a chance to take hold and cause an infection. Research shows that people catch colds and respiratory infections more often a few days after an event which makes them sad or upset. Other research (reviewed in Jemmott and Locke, 1984) shows that people who report being dissatisfied with life are more likely to have colds than those who report satisfaction. Yet more research shows that people who report feeling depressed or anxious are more likely to suffer from respiratory infections.

Another illness which can tell us about the competence of the immune system is that caused by the cold sore or herpes simplex virus. Cold sore sufferers have the virus HSV-1 present in their bodies all the time. The cold sore virus becomes active only when a person's defences are lowered. Cold sores have also been found to have a psychological basis. For example, Luborsky, Mintz, Brightman and Katcher (1976) report a study where young women entering nurse training were asked on each day to rate how happy they felt. On average, those students with cold sores felt more unhappy four days before the onset of the cold sore than four days after it. In addition, the researchers asked the nurse students to say whether they were typically happy or unhappy. Those who described themselves as typically unhappy had more occurrences of cold sores.

To sum up, there is a substantial body of research which shows that illnesses whose occurrence is largely controlled by the competence of the immune system are strongly affected by the mood of the person. In addition, daily mood changes have been shown to affect immune system activity as indicated through physiological measures (Stone et al, 1987). Thus, people who are unhappy, depressed and anxious are more likely to become ill because their immune systems are functioning less effectively.

However, it is not just mood which affects immune system functioning. There are some intriguing studies which show that expectations about future events also affect the immune system. Jackson et al (1960) gave subjects either a saline nasal spray or a nasal spray containing viruses. Subjects were told that the spray could be either saline or viral but were not told which sort they received. With both the viral and the saline solutions some people developed colds during the following two weeks. People receiving viral spray who expected to get a cold were more likely to do so (the people who developed colds did not have a prior history of more infections).

Other research (reviewed in Jemmott and Locke, 1984) shows that expectations resulting from hypnotic trances can also affect immune responses. For example, warts, which are removed naturally through activity of the immune system, can be treated through hypnosis for good but not for poor hypnotic subjects. Under hypnosis, good hypnotic subjects can alter the immune function of their skin, for instance reducing or increasing sensitivity to allergens, and this can be done selectively for one arm, for example, and not the other (e.g. Black, 1963). Contact dermatitis can also be altered through hypnosis and suggestion (Ikemi and Nakagawa, 1962; see also review in Hall, 1982).

Hypnosis (see chapter 7) operates through the mechanism of expectancy. Good hypnotic subjects are people who expect the hypnotic instructions to work: they have strong expectations about future events. Thus, people who are good hypnotic subjects may be more sensitive to the psychological effects of expectation than people who are poor hypnotic subjects.

The research described above shows that it is quite possible for a patient's beliefs about the likely course of an illness to have a physical effect on how that illness proceeds. People's expectations about their own illnesses may well be self-fulfilling because such expectations can actually alter the immune system in ways consistent with themselves.

Implications for nursing practice

Research into psychoimmunology has two kinds of implication for nursing practice. The first has to do with anticipating illness: people who have experienced a sad or unhappy event are more prone to infectious diseases. For example Bartrop et al (1977) report depressed lymphocyte activity in people who have suffered bereavement. People who are bereaved, who have ill or suffering relatives, or who are in some way unhappy are more likely to succumb to a variety of illnesses. Death is also more likely following the death of a spouse (Jones, 1987), though the extra likelihood of death is more marked in the first few weeks after the spouse's death. Flor et al (1987) found that the partners of patients in pain were also more likely to suffer from physical illness.

Thus, it seems that when people experience stressful family events such as pain in or bereavement of close relatives there is a drop in immunocompetence with an increased chance of illness and death. A nurse should assess a patient's psychological state as a way of finding out about his level of immunocompetence. The nurse should also find out about the relatives' psychological state following a stressful family event, and should be aware that they may need greater protection against infection (and possible resulting death) which arises from the poor function of the immune system.

The second implication of psychoimmunology for nursing is concerned with changing the patient's psychological state as a way of improving immunological function. Effective communication between the nurse and patient, which involves listening to the patient and providing the information he wants, can be an important factor in improving the patient's psychological state. Effective communication, however, is only a first step to satisfying the patient's needs. For example Brain and Maclay (1968) found that children whose mothers stayed with them in hospital (see chapter 6) were less likely to develop infections after tonsillectomy. At the time of carrying out the research, the important variable was thought to be whether mothers or nurses are more likely to spread infection. However, psychoimmunological research provides another interpretation of these results. It may have been that children whose mothers were present were happier and hence had more competent immune systems.

Lack of perceived control leads to learned helplessness and depression. As depression is an important factor in reducing immunocompetence (Baker, 1987) it is essential for nurses to use techniques which maximise the patient's own perception of control. Miller (1985) found more illness and death in long-stay elderly patients who received task-oriented care as opposed to individualised care (see chapter 1). When task-oriented care reduces the patient's perceived control over the environment, this lack of perceived control can lead to depression, and the depression can in turn lead to a lowering of immunocompetence.

- Mr Flanagan was confined to a wheelchair and suffered from considerable back pain. The community nurse called regularly to change the dressing on a venous ulcer on his leg. Mrs Flanagan was very upset by her husband's condition and reported to the community nurse that she often found it 'difficult to cope'. The community nurse not only treated Mr Flanagan, but also made time to talk to Mrs Flanagan who felt the community nurse was a 'real friend'. The nurse realised that Mrs Flanagan was at risk from infection, so was able to plan mechanisms for providing help under such circumstances. She was not only caring for the patient, Mr Flanagan, but also extending her care to the whole family. Moreover, the community nurse was both reacting to and anticipating illness.

The fact that psychological factors affect the immune system must be viewed from a holistic perspective. There are no grounds for abandoning cleanliness and antibiotics on the basis that an effectively operating immune system can deal with infection by itself. Whatever the psychological state of a patient, certain infections require external, biological intervention to put things right. However, one should also not lose sight of the fact that 'faith healing' does occur and that one mechanism by which it may operate is through changes in the immune system of a patient who believes in it.

CANCER

The term 'cancer' is used for a class of diseases which can be quite different in terms of aetiology and treatment. *Benign tumours* are overgrowths of normal tissue cells, which do not spread throughout the body. In *malignant tumours*, however, the mechanisms controlling growth are faulty and large numbers of abnormal cells are produced.

Cancer is a type of illness about which there is much misunderstanding in the general population. Opinions vary between the over-optimistic, i.e. that cancer is easily cured, to the over-pessimistic, i.e. that it is usually fatal. In fact improved use of surgery, chemotherapy, radiotherapy and bone marrow transplants have considerably improved the prognosis for a cancer sufferer. The likely outcome depends considerably on the particular type of cancer involved as well as on certain unknown or partially-known factors such as the patient's personality. At the time of diagnosis it is often quite difficult to predict the likely outcome so patients and their relatives are faced with the difficulty of coping with this uncertainty.

Patients and their relatives can also misunderstand the cause of cancer. First, cancer is not contagious, though some people may think erroneously that it is; it is worth pointing this out in case patients and their relatives think otherwise. Second, there is no strong evidence for a hereditary basis for cancer. Certain physical characteristics do make the person more prone to cancer and, to the extent that these physical characteristics are genetically determined, there is a hereditary element. But as a general rule patients should be reassured that the risk of cancer cannot be inherited.

The following cancers do, however, show a weak hereditary basis.

1. Daughters of mothers with breast cancer are slightly more at risk for developing breast cancer.

2. Fair skin, which is excessively sensitive to light, is more prone to developing skin cancer.

3. There is a hereditary condition (familial intestinal polyposis) in which polyps hang down into the colon, and can become irritated and develop into bowel cancer.

4. Retinoblastoma is a rare cancer of the eye found in young children which appears to have a hereditary basis.

What, then, is the cause of cancer? At the moment researchers do not know exactly what causes cancer, but quite a lot is known about the different factors which can predispose someone to develop cancer.

Cancers develop in two stages. The first stage involves the development of precancerous growths. These occur more readily in the presence of environmental agents called *carcinogens*. The second stage involves the transformation of the precancerous growths into active cancers. These growths do not necessarily change into cancers; whether they do so or not depends partly on the immune system, and the activity of the immune system, as described above, is affected by psychological factors.

Carcinogens

Carcinogens are substances which irritate body tissue or damage the genetic material in cells, thereby stimulating or allowing cells to reproduce rapidly and form precancerous growths. Of course, body tissue can be irritated in other ways: constant physical damage also irritates tissue and predisposes cells to form precancerous growths.

Carcinogens are both naturally-occurring and man-made. Naturally-occurring carcinogens include sunlight (which causes skin and lip cancers), radon gas emitted from granite rock and viruses such as the sexually transmitted virus harmless to men but which can cause cervical cancer in women. Man-made carcinogens are substances which have been manufactured for human use. These include tobacco products and substances such as benzidine which are used in certain industrial processes.

We are all exposed to one degree or another to carcinogens, but the extent to which a person comes in contact with carcinogens, both naturally-occurring and man-made, is in part affected by psychological factors. For example, people smoke and overexpose themselves to sunlight by choice. Reduced contact with carcinogens is an obvious way to reduce cancer in a population but there are two obstacles in getting people to avoid carcinogens. The first is purely educational. People need to be taught that excessive sunlight, tobacco products, asbestos and various other chemical products are carcinogenic, otherwise there is no reason for them to avoid these substances. The second obstacle is motivational: people need to not want to smoke or come in contact with other carcinogenic products. Chapter 3 describes some of the ways of presenting information which involves the likelihood of patient cooperation.

Smoking is a major cause of cancer. People smoke for many reasons: for example, as a way of coping with stress, as a tool for social interaction, and because it is enjoyable. Because of the many positive reasons for smoking, and because smokers are addicted to the nicotine in cigarettes, it is very difficult to persuade people to stop smoking. Indeed, many people who want to stop find it impossible. If a patient is unable to give up smoking completely, he or she will have a better chance of survival if smoking is discontinued periodically, for example, for one day of every week. People who persistently smoke (for example, who continue smoking during a cold) are more likely to develop lung cancer than those who allow their lungs periods of recovery (Lambley, 1986).

Lambley proposes, too, that there is a tendency for some people to be insensitive to their body's warning signals. Some people are sensitive to tissue irritants and avoid them or at least do not expose themselves to them all the time. Other people are less sensitive to irritants. People in the latter category have learned to 'over-ride' their own body's warning signals and are more prone to develop cancer. Lambley also suggests that cancers develop in specific sites of the body when people tend to ignore irritation in that area.

Lambley's idea of the relationship between self-monitoring and health receives support from other research. Suls and Fletcher (1985) used a questionnaire to divide a group of subjects into two groups: those who tended to be conscious of their own feelings and thoughts (the high self-conscious group) and those who were generally not conscious of feelings and thoughts (the low self-conscious group). Suls and Fletcher asked all subjects to keep a record of illness and of 'undesirable and uncontrollable life events' over a period of a month. The researchers found that there was no relationship between undesirable or uncontrollable life events and illness in the high self-conscious group but there was a relationship in the low self-conscious group. In the low self-conscious group, people who had experienced more negative life events tended to have more illnesses. The researchers conclude that self-attention is a 'stress-resistance resource', i.e. helps to guard against stress.

In general terms, then, people who are conscious of what their bodies and minds are trying to tell them tend to be healthier. Chapter 2 introduced the idea of nurses making 'exploratory' statements as a way of developing a therapeutic relationship and as a way of encouraging patients to think about and describe their feelings. This idea of self-exploration should not be limited to only the patient's mental state. As part of health education, the nurse should encourage patients to become aware of their own bodies as this is an important aspect of healthy living.

Cancer and the immune system

Contact with carcinogens is not sufficient to cause cancer. Not everyone who smokes develops cancer – as smokers often point out as a way of justifying their habit. Contact with carcinogens simply predisposes someone to develop cancer. As stated earlier, carcinogens irritate the body tissue, and groups of precancerous cells can form. Precancerous growths are probably constantly appearing but, in a healthy body, are removed by the body's own defence mechanism, the immune system. If precancerous growths are not removed they may develop into true cancers. One type of white blood cell seems primarily responsible for eliminating precancerous growths; this is called the natural killer cell.

Natural killer cell activity is affected by environmental and personality factors. Cancer is therefore more likely to occur in people who have particular sorts of experience and particular types of personality. Stressful life events have long been associated with the development of cancer (Sklar and Anisman, 1981). For example, cancer is more likely to develop in people who have been recently bereaved. However, it is often not the stressful event itself which causes the cancer, but the interpretation placed upon that event. People who react to stress by becoming depressed are more likely to develop cancer than those who react to stress by 'fighting it'. Among patients who have already developed cancer those who are 'fighting' their cancer have a much better prognosis than those who react to their condition with feelings of helplessness.

Derogatis (1986) finds that patients who succumb to cancer tend to be polite, coopera-tive and unable to express hostility. People who react to the news of their illness with a fighting spirit fare better than those who react with stoic acceptance.

Research relating to the 'difficult' patient was reviewed in chapter 4. The 'difficult' patient is often someone who does not passively accept an unsatisfactory situation but tries to do something about it, and appears uncooperative as a consequence. In that the 'difficult' patient is not reacting with feelings of helplessness, it would appear that he has a better chance of survival than the cooperative 'good' patient, a point confirmed by Derogatis' study.

Overall, the research seems to indicate that the depressive, helpless reaction to stress reduces the activity of the natural killer cells, which in turn reduces the body's capacity to deal with precancerous growths. The diagnosis of cancer is itself almost invariably highly stressful. It is therefore important when nursing patients with cancer to provide an optimistic, positive atmosphere where patients can be actively involved in fighting their cancer rather than slumping into a passive state of depression.

There are several companies which market 'health imaging' video films and audio-tapes which teach people how to imagine that their white blood cells are killing cancer or infectious cells. Patients with cancer have also been encouraged to play video games where they 'shoot down' cancer cells. One reason behind the effectiveness of these imaging techniques may simply be that they provide the patient with a framework of perceived control for fighting the cancer. Such techniques discourage feelings of helplessness by giving the patient something to do to try and make the cancer go away. Inevitably, the effectiveness of these techniques is likely to be affected by whether the patient believes health imaging to be a therapeutic procedure, just as faith healing may work purely through the expectation that the healer is effective.

There have been several research studies which have examined the personality characteristics of cancer-prone people (see reviews by Derogatis, 1986; Lambley, 1986). The cancer-prone personality is described by three traits: first, feelings of depression often occasioned by some unresolved loss; second, inability to express frustration and anger, i.e. the tendency to bottle up feelings; and third, weak interper-sonal relationships, for example with parents. Interestingly, the cancer-prone per-sonality shares much in common with the disease-prone personality identified by Friedman and Booth-Kewley (1987). Basically, people who are happy and relaxed tend to be healthier than people who are anxious, depressed and unhappy.

Lambley (1986) suggests that the personality characteristics which predispose someone to develop or be protected from cancer are affected by the way he is brought up. Children who are reared in a cold, impersonal atmosphere and who are discour-aged from expressing feelings such as grief will, as adults, be less able to express emotion and have poorer family ties. They will therefore be more likely as adults to develop personalities which predispose them to developing cancer. On the other hand, children who are brought up in a warm, supportive atmosphere where they are able to cry and express feelings are less likely to develop cancer when adult. Health education for cancer should start with parentcraft as parents play a vital role in the development of their children's personalities.

Patients with cancer may be treated with a combination of surgery, chemotherapy, radiotherapy and bone marrow transplantation. These medical interventions have their own psychological costs to the patient, including change of body image from surgery, as well as the physical results of nausea and vomiting which are often associated with chemotherapy and radiotherapy. Nausea and vomiting often get worse during treatment due to the effect of learning by association. Learning by association was first investigated by the Russian psychologist, Pavlov. In his famous experiment he rang a bell whenever he gave a dog food, and the dog salivated in response to the food. After a while, the dog salivated on hearing the bell ring even though no food was given. The bell and the act of salivation became associated through learning. In the case of patients with cancer, treatment often leads to nausea and vomiting. As a result aspects of the situation related to treatment (e.g. the hospital's smell, the treatment room or the staff) can become associated with nausea and vomiting. For this reason veteran patients will sometimes vomit before treatment actually begins.

Burish and Carey (1986) show that anxiety increases the learned vomiting response which occurs in cancer chemotherapy. That is, anxiety encourages people to learn to feel nauseous during chemotherapy and so they are more likely to be troubled by nausea and vomiting during the treatment. A good therapeutic relationship and provision of correct information helps reduce feelings of anxiety (see chapters 2 and 3). Thus, good psychological care by nurses is helpful for patients with cancer undergoing chemotherapy as it should indirectly reduce the feelings of nausea. Distraction has also been found useful in reducing nausea during the treatment of cancer, for example Redd et al (1987) found that if children with cancer played video games their nausea lessened. It is interesting to note that these two care techniques for reducing nausea, anxiety reduction and distraction, are also techniques which can be used when caring for patients in pain (see chapter 7).

CORONARY HEART DISEASE

The heart is a pump which forces blood round the body. The walls of the heart are made of muscle and this is supplied with oxygen from blood flowing through the coronary arteries. *Atherosclerosis* is a condition in which the arteries gradually narrow due to fatty deposits forming on the inside of the artery wall. These fatty deposits reduce blood flow and the oxygen supply to the heart muscle, and thus its efficiency.

Two major symptoms occur from the gradual narrowing of the coronary arteries and consequent reduction in oxygen supply. The first, known as *angina pectoris* is a pain felt in the chest, due to the heart muscle being starved of oxygen. Angina pain is often associated with physical exercise or emotional stress. Second, a heart attack or myocardial infarction occurs when a coronary artery becomes blocked, which can occur suddenly from a blood clot lodging in the artery or gradually by muscular spasm of the sclerosed vessel wall.

There is, however, a complicating factor. Post-mortem examinations of victims of lethal heart attacks show that they often have hearts that are physically 'too good to die'. It is not just deficits in the blood supply which cause death; electrical instability of the heart can also be fatal. Electrical activity in the heart normally starts in the sinoatrial node or pacemaker in the right atrium of the heart and spreads to the heart muscle, causing it to contract with a regular beat. However, the activity in the sinoatrial node may become irregular (arrhythmic). Additionally, especially in the first few hours after myocardial infarction, abnormal *ectopic* beats arise from the heart muscle itself and result in the heart contracting out of synchrony, i.e. different regions of the heart muscle contract independently of each other. The consequence of this lack of synchrony is that, although the heart muscle contracts, the heart no longer acts as an effective pump and death follows in a matter of minutes. Irregular heart beats which occur in the first few hours after a heart attack must therefore be controlled, and this can be done to some extent by drugs.

There are a number of factors which determine who suffers from coronary heart disease. People with high blood pressure or high levels of blood cholesterol have been found to be at risk for coronary heart disease. The high blood pressure puts an additional strain on the heart which has to pump against this pressure, and the high blood cholesterol level increases the risk of atherosclerosis. People who smoke are at greater risk of coronary heart disease, as are people who do not engage in physical exercise. Coronary heart disease also tends to occur in families, though to what extent this is genetic or caused by social factors is unclear.

One way of reducing coronary heart disease is to teach people to reduce their exposure to the risk factors. For example, the educational programme in the United States and Finland to reduce fat (cholesterol) intake and take exercise is thought to be responsible for the reduction in coronary heart disease in these countries in recent years. In fact, it seems that only some people need to reduce their cholesterol intake; others are able to metabolise it so that their blood cholesterol level is low irrespective of intake. Hence, knowledge of a patient's blood cholesterol level is useful when giving health advice about diet.

Education in self-care as a way of reducing coronary heart disease needs to overcome two obstacles. First, people must know what they should do and, second, they must want to do it. Avoiding cholesterol, taking exercise and giving up smoking all have their negative consequences and may not be engaged in for that reason. Ways of presenting information so as to maximise compliance with health care instructions are described in chapter 3.

In recent years two psychological risk factors have been found to be associated with coronary heart disease: These are 'Type A' personality and loneliness.

Type A personality

In the 1950s, Friedman and Rosenman, two Californian cardiologists were told by their secretary that their waiting-room chairs were getting worn down, but only on the front of the seats. It appeared that their patients were in a tremendous hurry to be seen and leave, and were sitting on the edge of their chairs. Friedman and Rosenman originally called this phenomenon the 'hurry sickness', which they later changed to the term 'Type A behaviour pattern' (Friedman and Rosenman, 1974). Research in the subsequent decades has generally (though not always) confirmed the idea that a particular type of personality (Type A personality) and type of behaviour increases the likelihood of coronary heart disease, whereas another type of personality (Type B personality) and way of behaving decreases the likelihood.

The Type A personality is ambitious, aggressive, competitive and impatient. Type A people react to obstacles by getting irritated or angry; they do not like wasting time. The Type A person is always in a hurry trying to achieve goals, but never has quite enough time to get everything done.

The Type B personality has an alternative way of coping. Type B people are more relaxed, easy going, readily satisfied and not continually driven to achieve. They are prepared to accept that things will not get done, without feeling anxious or upset.

The Type A personality or behaviour pattern constitutes a risk factor for coronary heart disease, and like any other risk factor it is possible to reduce it. Therapeutic and educational programmes can help people to change from a habitual Type A pattern of behaving which puts them at risk for coronary heart disease to one which puts them at less risk. Research has shown these therapeutic and educational programmes are effective in reducing coronary heart disease, at least for some people (Nunes, Frank and Kornfeld, 1987). Programmes designed to reduce Type A behaviour include some of the following techniques.

1. Education about Type A behaviour and coronary heart disease.

2. Relaxation techniques (see chapter 7).

3. Cognitive therapy, which is designed to change the Type A way of thinking into a Type B way of thinking. For example, the patient is advised to change the thought 'I have to get there quickly' into 'I am going fast enough'.

4. Imaging techniques, where the patient imagines that he is in a traffic jam or a confrontation with someone and mentally rehearses relaxed (Type B) ways of coping with the situation.

5. Role play of relaxed (Type B) coping strategies.

6. Emotional support where patients are encouraged to talk about their feelings in a sympathetic atmosphere.

Any patient who suffers a heart attack is likely to be anxious about his condition, particularly if he is of a Type A disposition. Research (Levine et al, 1987) shows that patients who are 'disengaged' from, i.e. withdraw from, the concerns and anxieties of the disease make a better recovery in the acute phase of coronary disease. However, such individuals show less compliance and require more rehospitalisation after discharge. The implication for nursing practice is that the nurse should encourage disengagement from worry in the acute phase of coronary disease, as the reduction in anxiety aids recovery. However, on discharge the nurse should emphasise the need to comply with self-care instructions to prevent a reoccurrence of coronary problems.

Although on discharge patients are usually given instructions about the amount of exercise they should attempt, sexual activity is often not referred to. Heart attack victims are often very worried about resuming such activity, because it increases heart rate and places stress on the heart. Problems can arise if patients are worried about the possibility of a heart attack or chest pain during sexual activity. It is important that the patient is given clear instructions about when he should resume sexual activity (which may or may not include sexual intercourse).

Loneliness

Single and widowed men and women have a greater risk of heart disease than those who are married (Jones, 1987). The considerable data supporting the idea that loneliness and lack of human contact contributes to heart disease is explored by Lynch (1977) in his book 'The Broken Heart'. Lynch argues that lack of love and human companionship is a contributor to heart disease, and that the expression 'dying of a broken heart' has a very real physical meaning in that the sadness occasioned by bereavement can cause heart attacks and death.

Lynch's own research (Lynch et al, 1974) shows how human contact can help in the care of patients following myocardial infarction. Such contact appears to have profound effects on how the heart functions. Physical contact can increase the flow of blood in the coronary arteries but, more importantly, it can reduce or completely eliminate irregular heart beats. These irregular beats, it will be remembered, are common in the hours following a heart attack and can lead to the heart muscle contracting out of synchrony, resulting in death.

Lynch's research shows that if a nurse holds the hand of a patient, even if the patient is in a coma, this action can slow the heart rate and reduce the number of irregular heart beats. Furthermore, contact is improved by the nurse talking to the patient, even though the patient is unable to reply. Physical contact and a warm, sympathetic style of care can thus have crucial effects on the recovery of people who have had heart attacks.

Lynch found that patients in a cardiac intensive care unit had a better chance of recovery if the nurse held the patient's hand and comforted him with the following kind of statement, the statement being individualised for the particular patient.

● (First name of patient), my name is (first name of nurse) and I am a nurse. I know you can't answer me when I talk to you even though you can hear me. That's because of your medication. You're receiving a drug called curare which has temporarily paralysed you so you are unable to respond in any way. The drug has also blocked your respiration, so there is a machine at your bedside breathing for you, which you may be able to hear. This medicine is an unpleasant but necessary part of your therapy, so please try to relax and bear with it. As I said before, the effect will only be temporary, and once the drug is discontinued you will be able to move as before. We will try to anticipate your needs, since you are at present unable to communicate them to us. There is always a doctor or nurse at your bedside, so please try not to worry. (From Lynch, 1977, p.143)

Implications for nursing practice

Below is a summary of the implications for nursing from the above account of coronary heart disease.

First, nurses should recognise that some people are more at risk of heart disease than others. The psychological factors associated with increased risk of heart disease are loneliness (either chronic or occasioned by bereavement or loss) and Type A behaviour.

Second, nurses should educate patients in order to reduce their risk of coronary heart disease. Such education includes reducing physical risk factors such as smoking and not taking exercise, but should also include information about psychological risk factors. For example, patients could be educated about Type A behaviour, particularly middle aged males who have a much higher incidence of coronary illness than women. For lonely patients having a pet can reduce feelings of isolation and, indeed, can protect against coronary illness.

Third, psychological care of coronary patients should have two main objectives, first, to reduce the patient's anxiety, and, second, to provide human contact and a warm sympathetic atmosphere for recovery: a good therapeutic relationship can save lives in coronary care.

THE MIND-BODY RELATIONSHIP IN PERSPECTIVE

The mind can affect the incidence and outcome of physical illness, and physical illness can affect the mind. The purpose of this section is to provide an overview of the mind–body relationship to enable the nurse to develop her own strategies in caring for patients with particular illnesses.

The mind affects the body in two ways. First, mood and expectation can have direct physiological consequences, for example, by altering the functioning of the immune system, the development of cancer and the functioning of the heart. Mood state can also affect many other physiological functions, in particular those relating to the autonomic nervous system. In fact, mood and expectation (which differ between people with different personalities) are related to a host of illnesses, and this has given rise to the idea of the 'disease-prone personality' (Friedman and Booth-Kewley, 1987), which includes the traits of anxiety, depression, and anger. Bearing this in mind, nurses should try to improve the mood states of patients in their care, in particular by trying to reduce anxiety, depression and anger.

A second way in which the mind affects the body is that choices regarding the way a person lives affects his physical health. Choices are made to smoke or drink excessive alcohol. Nurses have a health education role to play in trying to reduce the extent to which people engage in self-harming behaviours. Needless to say, simply telling people to stop smoking or telling them that they have a drink problem is unlikely to be effective (see chapter 3). Health education often involves giving personally-threatening information, and such information must be given in situations of unconditional positive regard so that the patient does not feel he is being reprimanded by an authority figure.

Of course, people may smoke or drink for other psychological reasons, for example as a way of avoiding anxiety or depression. Thus, behaviours which are self-harming at one level (e.g. smoking increases contact with carcinogens) may not be self-harming at some other level (e.g. the absence of depression maintains immunocompetence). The nurse must be aware that potentially harmful behaviours such as smoking, drinking, reckless driving and even dangerous sports are not carried out by the patient in order to kill himself, but for other reasons. There is always a temptation for health professionals to sit in judgment on those who engage in potentially self-harming behaviours, because the goals of these people are so different from the carer's goal of maintaining quality of life. Nurses should resist this temptation to judge those whom they believe are endangering their own lives.

Suicides and attempted suicides make up an important category of self-harming behaviour where there is a conscious attempt to end or endanger life. Researchers on suicide (Shneidman, 1980, 1985) have found that suicide is not an incomprehensible act of self-destruction. Instead, suicidal people have a way of thinking that brings them to the conclusion that suicide is the only solution to their problems. They often report unendurable psychological pain, and suicide is seen as a way of escaping that pain and ending consciousness. The pain often results from frustrated psychological needs, in particular love, achievement and trust. In searching for a solution, suicidal people show a 'constriction of options' where there seem only to be the options, 'Either all my problems go away or I commit suicide'.

Some patients who attempt suicide (typically by taking a drug overdose) appear to have apparently trivial reasons for trying to kill themselves, for example break-up with a boy-friend or low marks at school. However, what may be trivial to a mature nurse may not be trivial to a teenager. Because people have different needs, the nurse should not dismiss a patient who has attempted suicide as 'wasting everyone's time' simply because the patient's needs are different from her own. As shown earlier many illnesses, such as cancer and coronary illness, can result from self-harming behaviour. Attempted suicide is just an extreme example where the perceived benefits of self-harm outweigh the perceived benefits of health care. Schneider (1985) writes, 'While there are many pointless deaths, there is never a needless suicide'.

Some patients who attempt suicide simply do not wish to talk. They may find the experience of being in hospital just as psychologically painful as the events which caused their suicide attempt. However, if a patient wishes to talk, one useful counselling technique may help, particularly if the patient is going to be discharged without any professional counselling. The aim of this technique is to overcome the constriction of options which the suicidal person experiences. The nurse takes a sheet of paper and writes down, with the patient, all the options including all the ones which he finds unacceptable (typically, the only acceptable option is death). Then the patient is asked to rank these unacceptable options in order of preference, at the same time being told that the nurse accepts that he is not going to do any of these options. The very act of making such a list in a non-judgmental manner can help broaden the patient's options. By focusing on these other options, the patient may find that death is, in fact, less preferred than some other option.

Although mind can affect the incidence of and outcome of physical illness and death there is another way in which minds and bodies are related. The physical characteristics of the body can affect the mind. For example, patients on renal dialysis typicaily go through a 'honeymoon' period when treatment begins and they feel better, but then they experience feelings of anger and irritation that their lives are so constricted by the treatment. Patients who have stomas often feel anxious about odour and the fact that they may not be attractive to others. Women who have undergone mastectomies and hysterectomies may feel that they have lost a part of their femininity and sexuality and react with feelings of loss and depression. No two patients react to such psychologically distressing conditions in the same way. For some women, a hysterectomy is psychologically like losing an appendix (although after a hysterectomy there may be physical side-effects such as tiredness, back pain, constipation and dryness of the vagina). For other women, a hysterectomy leads to a total reappraisal of her role as a woman, and so may lead to psychological and sexual problems.

Psychological problems which result from physical illness must not be ignored, first, because a nurse should try to minimise psychological suffering and, second, because the psychological state which results from illness can spiral back and affect the illness. For example, suppose a woman has a mastectomy due to the discovery of malignant tissue in her breast. If that woman reacts to the mastectomy with feelings of depression and personal inadequacy when relating to others, her feelings may lead to a lowering of immunocompetence, in particular a reduction in natural killer cell activity. Thus, the psychological consequences of losing a breast may make a woman more susceptible to cancerous growths in other parts of her body. The mind–body relationship is two-way, and there can be cycles where psychological states lead to physical conditions and physical conditions alter psychological states.

Although through history it has appeared that the mind affects the body and the body affects the mind, modern views (Lambley, 1986; Hyland, 1985; Kirsch and Hyland, 1987) suggest that minds and bodies are just different perspectives on what is essentially a single unitary person. To illustrate this point, consider the finding that premature babies, once they leave intensive care units, show considerably better weight gain if they are massaged (Field, 1986). Is the massage affecting the babies' minds or their bodies? Clearly, massage affects people in ways which involve both the body and the mind.

At the beginning of this book it was suggested that nursing involves both psychological and physical care. However, the physical and psychological care are really not that separate. Whenever a nurse engages in physical care, she affects the whole person including his psychological state. Physical and psychological care are just descriptive categories. What the nurse actually does is to provide care.

SUMMARY

This chapter has focused on the mind–body relationship: the mind affects the body and the body influences the mind. The chapter is divided into four sections.

1. Psychological factors relating to the functioning of the immune system and the implications these psychological factors have for nursing care

2. Psychological factors relating to the development and treatment of cancer

3. Psychological factors relating to the development and treatment of coronary heart disease

4. The mind–body relationship in perspective

The overall finding is that people who are happy are less likely to get ill and more likely to recover from disease. Clearly, psychological care is important as a way of maintaining good physical health.

In addition, nurses should play an educational role where possible. Prevention is better than cure and self-care while healthy is a powerful tool for retaining good health.

Finally, this chapter dispels the myth of the biological model of illness. Patients should be cared for as whole people, not as bodies with diseases.

References

Baker G H B (1987) Psychological factors and immunity. *Journal of Psychosomatic Research,* **31**: 1–10.

Bartrop R W, Lockhurst E, Lazarus L, Kiloh L G and Penny R (1977) Depressed lymphocyte function after bereavement. *Lancet,* **i**: 834–836.

Benner S (1963) *From Novice to Expert.* Menlo Park, California: Addison-Wesley.

Black S (1963) Inhibition of immediate type hypersensitivity response by direct suggestion under hypnosis. *British Medical Journal,* **i**: 925–939.

Brain D J and Maclay I (1968) Controlled study of mothers and children in hospital. *British Medical Journal,* **i**: 278–280.

Burish T G and Carey M P. (1986) Conditioned aversive responses in cancer chemotherapy patients: theoretical and developmental analysis. *Journal of Consulting and Clinical Psychology,* **54**: 593–600.

Derogatis L R (1986) Psychology in cancer medicine: a perspective and overview. *Journal of Consulting and Clinical Psychology,* **54**: 632–638.

Engel G L (1977) The need for a new medical model: a challenge for biomedicine. *Science,* **196**: 129–136.

Field T (1986) Interventions for premature infants. *Journal of Pediatrics,* **109**: 183–191.

Flor H, Turk D C and Scholz O B (1987) Impact of chronic pain on the spouse: marital, emotional and physical consequences. *Journal of Psychosomatic Research,* **31**: 63–71.

Friedman H S and Booth-Kewley S (1987) The 'disease-prone personality': a meta-analytic view of the construct. *American Psychologist,* **42**: 539–555.

Friedman M and Rosenman R H (1974) *Type A Behaviour and Your Heart.* New York: Knopf.

Hall H R (1982) Hypnosis and the immune system: a review with implications for cancer and the psychology of healing. *American Journal of Clinical Hypnosis,* **25**: 93–103.

Hyland M E (1985) Do person variables exist in different ways? *American Psychologist,* **40**: 1003–1010.

Ikemi Y and Nakagawa S (1962) A psychosomatic study of contagious dermatitis. *Kyushu Journal of Medical Science,* **13**: 335–350.

Ishigami T (1919) The influence of psychic acts on the progress of pulmonary tuberculosis. *American Review of Tuberculosis,* **2**: 470–484.

Jackson G G, Dowling H F, Anderson T O, Riff L, Saporta J and Turck M (1960) Susceptibility and immunity to common upper respiratory viral infections–the common cold. *Annals of Internal Medicine,* **53**: 719–738.

Jemmott J B and Locke S E (1984) Psychosocial factors, immunologic mediation, and human susceptibility to infectious diseases: how much do we know? *Psychological Bulletin,* **95**: 78–108.

Jones D R (1987) Heart disease mortality following widowhood: some results from the OPCS longitudinal study. *Journal of Psychosomatic Research,* **31**: 325–333.

Kirsch I and Hyland M E (1987) How thoughts affect the body: a metatheoretical framework. *Journal of Mind and Behavior,* **8**: 417–434.

Lambley P (1986) *The Psychology of Cancer.* London: Macdonald.

Levine J, Warrenburg S, Kerns R, Schwarts G, Delaney R, Fontana A, Gradman A, Smith S, Allen S and Cascione R (1987) The role of denial in recovery from coronary heart disease. *Psychosomatic Medicine,* **49**: 109–117.

Luborsky L, Mintz J, Brightman V J and Katcher A H (1976) Herpes simplex virus and moods: a longitudinal study. *Journal of Psychosomatic Research,* **20**: 543–548.

Lynch J J (1977) *The Broken Heart; Medical Consequences of Loneliness.* New York: Basic Books.

Lynch J J, Thomas S A, Mills M E, Malinow K and Katcher A H (1974) The effects of human contact on cardiac arrhythmia in coronary care patients. *Journal of Nervous and Mental Diseases,* **158**: 88–89.

Miller A (1985) Nurse/patient dependency–is it iatrogenic? *Journal of Advanced Nursing,* **10**: 63–69.

Nunes E V, Frank K A and Kornfeld D S (1987) Psychologic treatment for the Type A behavior pattern and coronary heart disease. *Psychosomatic Medicine,* **49**: 153–173.

Redd W H, Jacobsen P B, Die-trill M, Dermatis H, McEnvoy M and Holland J C (1987) Cognitive/attentional distraction in the control of conditioned nausea in pediatric cancer patients receiving chemotherapy. *Journal of Consulting and Clinical Psychology,* **55**: 391–395.

Shneidman E (1980) *Voices of Death.* New York: Harper & Row.

Shneidman E (1985) *Definition of Suicide.* New York: Wiley.

Sklar L S and Anisman H (1981) Stress and cancer. *Psychological Bulletin,* **89**: 369–406.

Stone A A, Cox D S, Valdimarsdotirr H, Janorf L and Neale J M (1987) Evidence that secretory IgA antibody is associated with daily mood. *Journal of Personality and Social Psychology,* **52**: 988–993.

Suls J and Fletcher B (1985) Self-attention, life stress, and illness: a prospective study. *Psychosomatic Medicine,* **47**: 469–481.

10

The Art and Science

of Psychological Care

This book has focused on scientific research which is relevant to the provision of psychological care. This combination of nursing and psychology is certainly a science, but providing psychological care is something more than that: it is also an art.

This chapter is divided into three sections. The first section provides an overview of the science of psychological care as described in this book and shows how this science relates to the art of psychological care. The second section outlines how the art of psychological care may be developed through experience. The final section examines the giving of psychological care from the nurse's own perspective and in terms of her own satisfaction and personal development.

SCIENCE AND ART RELATED

The science of psychological care

The science of psychological care concerns rules of practice where the rules are based on sound, scientific evidence. For example, there is evidence that people can remember only a limited amount of the information which they are given at any one time. The rule of practice, therefore, is not to give patients too much information at once. Thus, the science of psychological care involves finding out and following those general rules which are best for patient care.

The rules of psychological care are generalisations, i.e. rules which apply most of the time although not necessarily all the time. The rules and suggestions which appear in earlier chapters of this book work most but not necessarily all the time. Each person is (a) in some respects like all other people, (b) in other respects like some other people, (c) and in yet other respects like no other person. The science of psychological care has to do with categories (a) and (b), because generalisations apply only to the general not to the unique. Adapting care to the unique features of a patient is more of an art than a science.

The art of psychological care

Psychological care is more than just following scientific rules. In implementing psychological care, the nurse brings her own unique characteristics to the nursing situation. What may be right for one nurse may not be right for another. Thus psychological care has a creative element where the nurse draws on the scientific evidence to formulate her own unique way of providing psychological care. Furthermore, a nurse may sometimes care for a patient with unique psychological characteristics that necessitate a form of care deviating from the normal rules of nursing practice. Recognising and caring for the unique aspects of a person is an art not a science.

The science of psychological care can be learned from a textbook such as this. The art of psychological care cannot be so learned because, by its very nature, an art is not a rule-following exercise. The art of psychological care starts from the scientific rules of psychological care but goes beyond those rules. The art of psychological care can be developed only through nursing experience and through the development of the nurse's personality.

Four major themes have appeared throughout this book. These themes are:

1. The holistic model of care
2. Communication
3. Differences between people
4. Self-determination

These four themes will now be reviewed in terms of both the science and the art of nursing. The aims are to show how the science of psychological care can be a starting point for the development of the art of psychological care and to alert the nurse to attitudes or modes of thinking which might be useful for developing this art.

The holistic model of care

The holistic model of care states that care requires attention to the physiological, psychological and social aspects of the patient. Two aspects of the holistic model have been emphasised: the effect of mind on body and the role played by relatives.

Mind and body: the science

The mind and body are different aspects of one and the same person. When the mind is unhappy, anxious or depressed there are corresponding changes in the way the body functions. And when the body suffers from disease there are corresponding changes in a person's mental state. The mind–body relationship is important for a scientific understanding of pain experience (see chapter 7) and for an understanding of the immune system, cancer, coronary disease and many other illnesses (see chapter 9). The mind–body relationship is also highlighted by research which shows that the style of nursing can affect physical recovery (see chapters 1 and 7). The mind–body relationship is relevant to research which shows that the presence of a parent can reduce infection and pain experience in hospitalised children (see chapters 6 and 7).

Mind and body: the art

Although this book has dealt exclusively with psychological care, the division between psychological and physical care is artificial. The mind and body act together and psychological and physical care should not be treated as being two unrelated categories. If psychological and physical care are treated as different there is the risk that one sort of care will be given priority over the other in a rigid and inflexible manner. In particular there is the risk that a nurse may focus on physical care to avoid the often demanding aspects of psychological care.

The art of understanding the mind–body relationship means having an awareness of how the physical and psychological aspects of a person interact, and being sensitive to the implications of any nursing action on each unique patient who is both mind and body.

Relatives: the science

People become patients when they are ill, but they still remain people who have relatives, friends and interests. Relatives (particularly parents, see chapters 6 and 7) are important because they care for patients in hospital as well as caring for patients when they return home. However, relatives are important not only as carers but also as people who themselves need care. The psychological suffering of carers can be considerable, particularly when their loved ones are in pain, in a life threatening condition, dying or dead (chapters 8 and 9), and relatives can be at increased risk from physical illness and death. Such psychological and physical suffering can be reduced through nurses caring for relatives, not just for the patients signed on to a ward.

Relatives: the art

A nurse should try to understand the psychology of a patient not as an isolated individual but as a member of a particular family. The patient's family is a unique collection of individuals who have unique relationships with each other. The nurse needs to attend to the relationships between different family members as a way of finding out about their unique needs.

Communication

The science

Communication is the tool of psychological care. It is needed to understand what patients think and feel and to develop a therapeutic relationship (see chapter 2). Communication is also needed to give patients information (see chapter 3) which enhances their self-care. Different communication rules are appropriate for different nursing contexts, such as caring for the elderly (see chapter 5) or for children (see chapter 6). Indeed, just about every chapter in this book describes some specific communication rule.

The art

The art of communication starts from the assumption that each nurse is unique. And because of this uniqueness, what one nurse should say is not necessarily suitable for another nurse. To be good at communicating, the nurse needs to feel comfortable about the way she is saying something. If she does not feel comfortable, what she says will easily sound insincere. The examples given in earlier chapters are only pointers to indicate the general effect a nurse should try to achieve. These examples should not be followed slavishly, but, instead, the nurse should try to explore how she may use her own natural style of communicating to its best advantage.

The art of communication develops through practice. When a nurse starts training she will tend to focus on herself during a conversation. She may think, 'Am I saying the right things? Am I engaging in the right level of eye contact?' A more experienced nurse communicator, however, carries out these rules without thinking, rather like an experienced cyclist does not need to think how to keep his balance. When the skills of communication are automatic the nurse is then able to focus not on herself but on the patient. It is only through detailed attention to what the patient is saying and how he is saying it that a nurse can use communication creatively to mesh her unique characteristics with those of the patient.

Differences between people

The science

In psychology the topic of personality is the scientific study of differences between people, specifically ways in which people are unlike some people but like others. An important theme in a number of chapters in this book is that individual differences are important to patient care. For example, patients experience pain and cope with pain in different ways (see chapter 7), people react to old age and retirement in varying manners (see chapter 5), people have diverse informational needs (see chapter 3) and explain the causes of things that happen in different ways (see chapter 4).

Although personality is clearly important from the point of view of individualising care, a nurse is not able to distribute personality questionnaires to patients. She often has to make a common sense assessment of personality, and the science of person perception (see chapter 4) shows how easy it is to make errors in judging another's personality.

The art

A nurse uses person perception as the starting point for individualising patient care. The art of person perception is the skill of arriving at personality assessments which are as accurate as possible and it also involves knowing when the nurse is in a position to make an assessment and when she is not. Person perception is open to bias.

The art of person perception is closely related to the art of communication. It is only through effective communication with a patient that a nurse can understand and so assess the patient's distinctive mode of psychological functioning. And, like the art of communicating, the art of understanding is improved with practice because, to understand, it is necessary to focus on the patient, not oneself or the ward routine.

Self-determination

The science

If people feel they have no control over what is happening, this can lead to various psychological deficits (see chapter 1). Furthermore, feelings of helplessness are associated with increased sensation of pain, poor physical recovery and poor health (see chapters 7 and 9). The ability of people to choose for themselves and determine their own lives is clearly crucial to both psychological and physical well-being. However, self-determination is not without its negative side. People freely choose to expose themselves to carcinogens through smoking, and they sometimes choose to end their own lives (see chapter 9).

The art

The art of self-determination is the art of balance: balance between the patient's need for self-determination and the nurse's wish to protect and care for the patient. For example, a nurse may need to balance the effects of giving a patient with senile dementia some control and thus risking self-harm, or taking that control away and thereby exacerbating the developing symptoms of dementia. Alternatively, the nurse may need to balance between the patient's idea of how care should be provided and the nurse's own idea about what is the best form of care for the patient. Clearly, there are times when a patient's own ideas of care are impractical or dangerous, and the nurse must assess whether the damage caused by preventing self-determination is worse than the damage caused by allowing it. Sometimes a patient's inappropriate ideas are the result of misinformation (see chapter 3) and can be handled from that perspective. There are also times (such as the shock stage of bereavement) when a patient is cared for best by being told what to do rather than by being given a choice. In providing psychological care, there is an art in deciding when to encourage or discourage self-determination, and an art in deciding the limits to which it is safe or practical to allow self-determination. And there is also an art, if those limits have been reached, in preventing self-determination in a way which is least psychologically distressing for the patient. The art of self-determination is one of balance and compromise.

DEVELOPING THE ART OF PSYCHOLOGICAL CARE

The art of psychological care involves attention to and perceptiveness of the details which are relevant to providing effective psychological care. Attention and perceptiveness cannot be taught through rules; they come about through experience and are the characteristic of the expert nurse (Benner, 1984), that is a nurse who has well-developed skills both in the art and science of psychological care.

Psychological care is a skilled activity and a useful way to understand how psychological care is improved with experience is to consider how other skilled activities are learned, such as learning to ride a bicycle or learning to play the violin.

When teaching someone to ride a bicycle, the first thing to do is to give them rules, for example, 'Turn the handle bars in the direction in which you feel yourself falling'. Nevertheless, however well one knows this rule of steering, it may still not be possible to keep balance. The rider has to practise until the rule becomes automatic. There are two differences between the experienced cyclist and the learner. First, the experienced cyclist is perceptually sensitive to balance. Second, the reaction of turning the handle bars to counteract falling comes more quickly and can be done without conscious awareness. Both the greater perceptivity to balance and the rule-following become automatic, rather than needing conscious direction.

Thus, when a nurse becomes experienced in the provision of psychological care, she becomes more perceptually aware of the information which she receives from the patient, and she acts on that information more quickly. Furthermore, the better perceptivity and rate of action occur without conscious awareness: the nurse just 'feels' that her action is right, just as the cyclist 'feels' that he knows how to keep his balance.

However, there is another aspect to the expert provision of psychological care which is best illustrated with the example of learning to play the violin. When someone learns to play the violin, the first step is to learn the simple rules for playing notes. The student violinist learns to hold the bow in a particular way and to press on the strings with the fingers of his left hand. At the next stage of proficiency, the student learns to put notes together to make a melody. At this second stage, the student's goal has actually changed from note-making to melody-making. In the final or expert stage in violin playing, the violinist no longer tries to play a melody, but tries to provide a good interpretation of a melody. Again the focus has changed, from melody-making to interpretation of melody. Of course, the expert violinist still plays notes and still plays melodies but his focus of attention has shifted.

This kind of shift in attention can also be found in the nurse who is an expert at providing psychological care (Benner, 1984). After learning the rules of psychological care, and when those rules are being carried out automatically, the expert nurse shifts her focus of attention from rule-following to some higher-level goal of providing effective patient care. At this higher level, the nurse can achieve objectives which cannot be realised from rule-following. By having an overall perspective and objective, the nurse is able to focus on the patient. For example, she can assess the balance between self-determination and self-harm, because her goal is not rule-following but that of providing effective patient care. The expert nurse is able to come to a decision in a situation where rule-following is not enough.

How, then does experience help in developing a nurse's skill in providing psychological care? There are three aspects of the art of psychological care which may be developed through experience. First, experience helps perceptivity: an experienced cyclist has a better sense of balance, an experienced violinist has a better sense of pitch and tone. An expert nurse has greater perceptivity for communication and for assessing individual differences, for example, she is better able to read the signals which a patient is sending. In particular, the expert nurse is better able at putting together signals from different channels. This increased sensitivity often occurs at an unconscious level. Thus, the expert nurse may report, 'I had a feeling he wasn't happy, though I don't know why'. Sometimes, an expert nurse will report her perception as a 'gut reaction', for example, by saying, 'Something just bothered me about Mr Cook; he just didn't seem to be talking in the way I expected'.

A second feature of experience is that the nurse can follow rules without having to think about them. Consequently, she is more effective and can do more things at once. Someone learning to ride a bicycle cannot pedal and hold a conversation at the same time, but an experienced cyclist can ride and talk. When nursing activities become highly practised the nurse has spare mental capacity to do other things at the same time. The expert nurse can therefore follow several channels of action simultaneously, and carry them out more quickly than the novice.

A third and final feature of experience is that the nurse has an overall perspective which allows her to prioritise rules and also to break rules if they do not fit in with the overall pattern which she is trying to achieve. The overall perspective of the expert nurse involves her ability to perceive patients and their families as having interrelated goals, her ability to perceive the relationship between the psychological and physiological aspects of a person, and the ability to strike a balance between self-determination and other factors. The expert nurse is employing the rules of psychological care but has a higher-level goal which involves integration between the different rules.

Of course, not everyone who learns the violin becomes an expert. Not everyone is able to stop trying to make a melody and instead focus on interpreting the melody. In the same way, not all nurses who have experience as nurses develop expertise in psychological care. Indeed, learner nurses with their natural experience of people may sometimes have more expertise than experienced nurses (Crotty, 1985). At least one factor will affect whether a nurse becomes an expert in psychological care, and this is whether she wants to or not.

An expert nurse is a nurse who is willing to learn through experience. She is always learning, and it is this capacity to learn which distinguishes mere experience from expertise. Due to the uniqueness and complexity of people there is always something to learn about them. There is always something to be discovered about psychological care, and that applies both to the science and to the art of such care.

PSYCHOLOGICAL CARE: THE NURSE'S PERSPECTIVE

Switching into 'psychological-care mode'

One of the suggestions of reversal theory (see chapter 4) is that people switch between 'modes', and when they are in one particular mode, their way of behaving may be very different from when they are in some other mode. Providing psychological care can be thought of as a mode, and people can switch into the psychological-care mode.

In general nursing, it is not possible to be in psychological-care mode all the time as psychological care takes time, and there are occasions when the nurse does not have the time to engage in such behaviour. For example, in an emergency situation like a cardiac arrest, the nurse may need to take very rapid action. There may be no time to talk except in relation to the physical care which is being used to resuscitate the patient. In other emergencies, e.g. during a heart attack, the nurse may give valuable psychological support by simply holding the patient's hand.

In some instances where there is no time pressure, the patient may not want psychological care. Some people simply do not wish nurses to explore their personal and private lives. There is thus an art in knowing when and when not to provide psychological care.

A nurse who analyses her own psychological state will be aware of switching in and out of the psychological-care mode. Often this switching is caused by some change in the situation. For example, a nurse may react to an emergency by switching out of psychological-care mode until the emergency is over, when the reduced time pressure means that time can be spent talking to the patient and relatives. Alternatively, a nurse working in a special care baby unit may switch from dealing with monitors into a psychological-care mode when she realises that a mother wishes to talk about her baby. Although such changes are often governed by the situation, it is useful to develop the skill of switching in and out of psychological-care mode. The ability to move into other modes is important in two situations: relaxing after finishing work and dealing with other (and often senior) colleagues at work.

Relaxing

Nursing is an emotionally demanding job, for example a patient's death can be very distressing for nurses. These feelings of distress should not be resisted, although they should be managed by aiming for controlled emotional involvement. In particular, the nurse's display of emotion can help bereaved relatives. However, a nurse may have to deal with death quite regularly and, at the end of her period of duty, the nurse has to go and face her own life, and perhaps her own husband and children. The ability to switch out of the emotionally-charged patient-centred mode when returning home helps prevent 'burn out' from these very intense emotions. Nurses use different techniques for switching out of the patient-centred mode. Some nurses are naturally able to go home and completely forget about their work, whereas others find it helpful to talk to others about their experiences, and to enter a 'being cared for' rather than a 'carer' mode. Support groups are particularly valuable in helping nurses gain the help they need although some nurses, who are so used to giving help to others, find it difficult to ask for help for themselves; and some nurses who are used to helping patients do not think it necessary to help nurses. Nurses, however, do have important needs of their own and cannot operate effectively if they are unhappy in their jobs. In particular, nurses will not be effective in the art of psychological care if their own psychological state is unsatisfactory.

Dealing with colleagues

In order to form a therapeutic relationship, a nurse must not be assertive. She must listen and attend to what the patient is saying. However, it is quite wrong to be unassertive all the time: there are times when the nurse needs to stick up for herself and be professionally assertive. For example, when dealing with management personnel, a senior nurse may need to be assertive to maintain adequate staffing levels. A junior nurse may need to be assertive to doctors or senior nurses to ensure that a patient receives the right sort of care. Nurses need to be assertive when taking the role of a patient's advocate, i.e. helping the patient achieve what he wants.

It is difficult to be both assertive and unassertive at the same time, but a nurse needs to be able to switch between these two modes of interacting with people. Previous chapters of this book have concentrated on the unassertive mode of interacting, but below are some techniques which can emphasise assertiveness.

Assertiveness

Successful assertiveness often involves an attitude of psychological distancing from the other person concerned. This distancing includes not worrying about whether the other person likes you or not. To be assertive, it is also necessary to believe in what you are saying, and so it is best to focus attention on the argument, not on the other person. To be assertive but not aggressive one should respect the other person's point of view but not change one's views from what one believes to be right. There are a few practical tips which can be given.

Assertive people do a lot of talking. If another person tries to 'butt in' and the nurse wishes to keep talking, she should raise her voice and avoid eye contact (the latter being a non-verbal signal that she is going to continue speaking).

If someone expresses a view different from the nurse's own, lack of compromise can be expressed through statements such as 'I see and understand why you say X, but I know that I am right in saying Y' or, 'We must agree to disagree on this point'. If the nurse cannot afford to 'agree to disagree' a useful alternative is the 'scratched record technique' i.e.:

- *Nurse:* Mr Davies tells me he must go home.
  Sister: I'm afraid he can't.
  Nurse: Mr Davies tells me he must go home.
  Sister: Well he can't until the doctor says so.
  Nurse: I am sorry, but Mr Davies tells me he must go home.
  Sister: Well, you could ring Dr Adams.
  Nurse: OK, I'll go and do that.
  (The nurse rings Dr Adams who says that it is perfectly acceptable for Mr Davies to go home.)

If the nurse does not want to answer the question she was asked, she can reply to some other question: politicians often use this technique when they are posed difficult queries. Alternatively, to avoid answering a question it is possible to ask another one in return (e.g. 'Why do you find it necessary to ask that?'). In particular, it is a good ploy not to answer personal questions as these can signal the use of a personal attack to keep the speaker quiet.

Research (Moscovici, 1976) shows that members of a minority are more likely to alter the majority's opinion if they are consistent in what they say and do, and if they give the impression that they are confident that they are right. However, if too extreme a position is taken this can be counter-productive as it alienates others. One can compromise slightly, but only slightly, away from the position being adopted by the majority.

Finally, when in a minority, it is best to use information as a basis for trying to change other people's opinions as a rational approach is in many instances more effective than simply being awkward. A useful strategy when trying to win an argument is to research the topic beforehand and argue the case as scientifically and dispassionately as possible.

On studying this list of techniques for being assertive, the reader may feel that assertive people are not very companionable. Indeed, the technique of being assertive is the reverse of what has been suggested in this book for dealing with patients. Being assertive does not help to develop a therapeutic relationship, although being assertive on a patient's behalf when acting as his advocate can. Nevertheless, there are occasions when assertiveness is essential, and a skilled nurse should be able to recognise when assertiveness is professionally necessary, and be able to switch into assertiveness mode to deal with the situation.

Nursing and personal development

People are affected by their careers. However, people carry out the same task in various ways so a particular job may affect different people differently. Nurses can choose to nurse in many different ways. Each nurse chooses whether and how often she switches into the psychological-care mode of nursing, and it is this, among other, choices, which makes nursing a profession rather than just a job.

If a nurse emphasises psychological care in her nursing she will develop her own psychological skills, skills which she can then use in other situations. These skills are numerous; they involve the ability to understand people, to form warm, caring relationships with others, to help others to achieve their goals, and to influence others. By contrast, if psychological care is not delivered a nurse does not develop those particular psychological skills or their associated personality characteristics. The nurse who does not deliver psychological care may develop other skills, but she will not develop that deep ability to empathise with others which has always been the hallmark and attraction of nursing. The way she chooses to nurse will affect who she becomes in 10 years' time; it affects her just as it affects the patients for whom she cares.

One final important point: a nurse who finds her way barred in the rewarding task of providing psychological care should not give up hope, as situations and people change. She should continue developing her skills and caring for her patients. The nursing profession always needs good nurses.

References

Benner S (1963) *From Novice to Expert*. Menlo Park, California: Addison-Wesley.
Crotty M (1985) Communication between nurses and their patients. *Nurse Education Today,* **5**: 130–134.
Moscovici S (1976) *Social Influence and Social Change*. London: Academic Press.

Index